Understanding Traumatic Stress

DR NIGEL C. HUNT
and
DR SUE McHALE

sheldon **PRESS**

To Jack and Conor

First published in Great Britain in 2010

Sheldon Press
36 Causton Street
London SW1P 4ST
www.sheldonpress.co.uk

British Library Cataloguing-in-Publication Data
A catalogue record for this book is available from the British Library

ISBN 978–1–84709–056–0

1 3 5 7 9 10 8 6 4 2

Typeset by Fakenham Photosetting Ltd, Fakenham, Norfolk
Printed in Great Britain by Ashford Colour Press

Produced on paper from sustainable forests

Contents

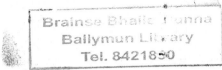
Preface

People who go through terrible life-threatening events, whether they relate to war, sexual abuse or rape, car accidents or natural disasters, can have serious psychological problems, ranging from nightmares and flashbacks, through physical responses and illness, to problems with experiencing emotions and being unable to have loving relationships. Traumatic events are shattering events, where everything you hold dear can break down. An experience of rape can mean that you are unable to trust anyone; war shows that people can behave in awful ways, and natural disasters such as earthquakes or tsunami show that even the natural world can be dangerous. If you have been through a life-threatening experience, you may well have changed your outlook on life fundamentally. For some, this change can be very damaging, and have long-lasting effects on both yourself and your family and friends.

This book is based on our research and experience over the last couple of decades working with people who have been through such experiences. Research shows that while everyone responds differently, there are some common responses. Traumatic events can lead to cognitive, emotional and behavioural effects. Cognitive effects are concerned with memories of the event and how your beliefs about the world and about people can be changed; emotional effects are to do with the fear, horror or helplessness that you feel after an event; and behavioural effects might include feeling nervous and jumpy, or being aggressive because of the traumatic event.

There are many ways to help someone who is traumatized. In many cases, people help themselves, by talking about what has happened to others, or by thinking it through or by writing about it. Often though, people need professional help from psychologists, therapists or counsellors. However this help is provided, whether by yourself or by a professional, it always involves trying to make sense of the traumatic event, trying to understand why someone acted as they did, or why you acted as you did.

This book aims to help both people who are traumatized and their friends and family to understand the symptoms associated with traumatic stress. For the people who are traumatized, the first stage of getting better is to understand their thoughts and memories. For family members or friends, it is just as critical to know why people act the way they do and say what they are saying, as the most important help that anyone can get is from his or her family and friends.

We hope the book will help you deal with traumatic experiences, whether these are your own or those of someone you love; but if the problems are very serious, it is important that help is sought from an appropriate professional, such as a clinical psychologist.

We would like to thank everyone who has helped out with this book. As we said above, social support is the most important kind of help anyone can get, so we would like to thank our family and friends; and also the people at Sheldon Press who have helped us through the process of preparing the book for publication.

About the authors

Dr Nigel C. Hunt is an academic psychologist – Associate Professor at the Institute of Work, Health and Organisations, University of Nottingham. He is also Reader in Traumatic Stress Studies at the University of Helsinki, Finland. He obtained his PhD at the University of Plymouth, entitled, 'The long-term psychological effects of war experience'. Since then he has written several books and numerous articles in academic journals and elsewhere, mostly on the subject of traumatic stress. He conducts research with war veterans and other traumatized people in a variety of contexts and in different countries.

Dr Sue McHale is Senior Lecturer in Biological Psychology at Sheffield Hallam University. She obtained her PhD at the University of Plymouth, and has interests in stress, coping and emotion, and in the effects of drugs on behaviour. She has written many articles in academic journals and elsewhere.

Dr Hunt and Dr McHale have written one book and several academic articles together, mainly on memory and on the psychosocial impact of alopecia.

Note to the reader

This is not a medical book and is not intended to replace advice from your doctor. Consult your pharmacist or doctor if you believe you have any of the symptoms described, and if you think you might need medical help.

1

Introduction

Jason

Jason returns home from the fighting in Afghanistan. In previous wars, he would have been greeted with flags and banners proclaiming his heroism, a true welcome home to the hero who had protected his country against the enemy that endangered its survival, but in this war there is no such welcome, only the depressing normality of civilian life. Jason is debriefed and is then given leave. He returns to his wife and there is happiness in being reunited. Jason decides to leave the army and get civilian work. This decision is made partly because he wants to spend more time with his wife and children, and they want to spend more time with him, and partly because he was not happy with his experiences in Afghanistan. He had seen things that bothered him – not too much, but they sometimes kept him awake at night.

For the first few months Jason is happy. He has a loving family and he has a job – not necessarily the job he wanted, but it brings in the money. Over time, however, he starts drinking more. He seeks out his old mates from the army, and starts spending more time with them and less time with his wife and children. His wife begins to get upset about this. When she confronts him, they start arguing. This makes him go out drinking even more. Eventually, he starts being late for work. When he does get there he causes trouble, and in the end he is sacked. Once unemployed, he feels he has no one to turn to but his mates in the pub. In the end his wife can't take any more and leaves him. He has no family and no job, and the pressures become too much. Up to this point the ex-soldier has not thought too much about the war; now his memories return with a vengeance. He gets depressed, he has nightmares, he has flashbacks and thinks he is back in Afghanistan.

Traumatic stress is not a simple disorder. It is not like the common cold or simple depression; it is not a straightforward set of symptoms that are the same in everyone who is traumatized. There are many different ways a person can respond to a traumatic event. Post-traumatic stress disorder (PTSD) does not just appear and then, with treatment, hopefully disappear. In many cases it comes on gradually and, as in the case of Jason described above, it may not be noticed for a long time. Other factors play a large part. For Jason, there were issues about civilian life, his family, drinking and other factors that came into play as part of the build-up to the PTSD. It may not be until many months, sometimes years, have passed that a person develops PTSD. It may be difficult for people to recognize at first, as a person's behaviour may appear to be the result of other things. This is one of the difficulties of the disorder.

Kate

Kate is returning home from a night out when she is attacked and raped. It is a particularly vicious attack and she ends up hospitalized. When she is released from hospital and returns home to her parents' house, she immediately goes to her room and locks herself in, refusing to talk to anyone. With great difficulty her parents get her to eat something; she will rarely talk to them, and she will say nothing about the attack. She doesn't go out with her friends, and generally refuses to see them when they visit her. She will not see boys at all. This behaviour goes on for some months before her parents persuade her to go for treatment. During this period Kate has had constant nightmares, repeated nightly showings of all the details of the attack. During her waking hours she thinks constantly about what happened, running the details through her mind, blaming herself for the attack, thinking that she should have avoided it. She is ashamed of herself. At first she constantly washes herself to try and become clean again. She will not look into a mirror because she cannot look into her own eyes. She does not work and she is fearful of any social relationships. She is at the same time anxious and depressed.

This is classic PTSD, the symptoms resulting from a single traumatic episode that has fundamentally damaged Kate's view of herself, other people and the world. It is said that people generally think well of themselves and others, regarding the world as by and large a good place, but that traumatic incidents such as rape fundamentally damage that belief system. The person who is raped sees that people can be bad, that the world is a bad place, and believes, 'I do not know how to behave properly if I allow such things to happen to me.' Kate cannot trust anyone any more, and feels guilty for not being able to personally stop the attack. Treatment is often at least partly about being able to restore one's faith in self, others and the world.

Post-traumatic stress disorder

Post-traumatic stress disorder (PTSD) has a traumatic history. The construct itself was not introduced into the psychiatric manuals until 1980, but the history of the subject goes back long before then. Famous figures such as Sigmund Freud, Marcel Breuer, Pierre Janet and Jean-Martin Charcot were discussing the subject in the late nineteenth century, but even before that it had been recognized that traumatic events such as war, fire or train crashes could cause serious psychological problems in people. We can explore diaries, journals and literature and find that throughout history there are accounts of such problems – though we often need to beware of how we interpret what people wrote many years ago, because the meaning of words does change, and terms such as 'traumatic stress' were unknown before the late nineteenth century.

One of the first well-known accounts that describe the psychological consequences of war is Homer's *Iliad*. Here, around 800 BC, Homer describes the experiences of Achilles, a general who is part of the besieging forces at Troy as the Greeks try to defeat the Trojans and return the beautiful Helen to Greece. Jonathan Shay, a psychiatrist from the USA with extensive experience of treating US veterans of the Vietnam War, noted that many of the symptoms described by Homer were similar to those experienced by the Vietnam veterans returning home to the USA after fighting. Indeed, Shay suggested – and we strongly support this idea – that our understanding of traumatic stress would be improved by the reading of Homer and other literary material, as it also describes aspects of the psychological and behavioural responses to war that are not covered by PTSD. At the end of the book, we provide a reading list if you are interested in following this further.

If we move forward a few hundred years to the battle of Marathon between the Persians and the Greeks, Herodotus describes how an Athenian soldier collapsed in battle. When he was found afterwards there was no trace of a wound, but his legs would not work and he was blind. We could suggest that this was an hysterical reaction to the terrors of war. He could not bear to see what was happening in the midst of battle so he shut his mind to it, and he could not bear to take part so his legs failed him. Herodotus states that the soldier never again learned to see. While Herodotus is not to be trusted as an historian, this sort of account is likely to have an element of truth, as similar accounts of reactions to war were reported by psychiatrists in the late nineteenth century and during the First World War.

We can trace similar descriptions of trauma throughout history, showing that it is not just a recent phenomenon. Instead, it is more helpful to look at how psychologists and psychiatrists have described these reactions. Most examples we have are war-related. We have always known that some troops – understandably – cannot cope with the horror of battle.

Up until the end of the nineteenth century – and well into the twentieth century – most people thought that psychological symptoms of traumatic events had physiological causes. In the US Civil War in the 1860s, it was thought that the cause of breakdown in battle was a weak heart. In the First World War it was thought that such breakdown was caused by microscopic injuries caused by shell fragments or shrapnel – hence the term 'shellshock'. This period from the US Civil War to the First World War saw some profound changes in the way we think about traumatic stress. And here we return to European psychiatrists such as Charcot, Freud and Janet.

We know Freud as the father of psychoanalysis. While he did not invent the unconscious, he certainly popularized it and with it created a sophisticated model of personality and the mind that appealed to people in Europe before and after the turn of the twentieth century. During the 1880s and 1890s Freud worked with Charcot, Breuer and others on understanding the reactions people have to traumatic events, and developed a theory relating to the relationship between the mind and behaviour which dominated much of psychology for decades. At the same time, Pierre Janet was working on a theory of traumatic stress that was more concerned with consciousness than with the unconscious. Janet suggested that after a traumatic event people develop traumatic memories (see Chapter 4) that need to be resolved into narrative memories, either through treatment or through some other means. As we shall see in Chapters 4 and 6, Janet was thinking ahead of his time. It can be argued that the development of abnormal psychology was delayed because the world decided that Freud's approach was more valid than that of Janet. We focused on the unconscious, rather than addressing consciousness.

During the First World War there were significant advances in our understanding of traumatic stress. In Austria, Freud worked with Austrian patients, and various teams worked with British and Allied psychiatric casualties. As mentioned above, the term 'shellshock' was derived from the view then held that physiological damage underlies psychological trauma, but it was during the First World War that people began to recognize that the cause was psychological: that something can be so horrific, terrifying and life-threatening that it can cause profound mental changes – in other words, traumatize someone. It was also during the First World War that the first treatment principles were applied. These were known as PIE: proximity, immediacy and expectancy. Traumatized soldiers were to be treated as close to the front line as possible (proximity), as soon as they displayed symptoms (immediacy), and always knowing that they would be sent back to their front line unit (expectancy). This last was important: they were never to think of themselves as casualties, injured victims, but just as people who were tired of fighting and needed a rest.

In the Second World War the USA forgot these rules and initially sent their psychiatric casualties back with the physically wounded. This led to a severe depletion of combat units, so the policy was quickly changed. The British started with a very small psychiatric unit in the Second World War, but William Sargent, a psychiatrist, saw the troops returning from Dunkirk and realized that they needed psychiatric help, not just rest and recuperation. He helped develop sophisticated psychiatric services for the British armed forces.

The attitude towards traumatized troops changed between the First and Second World Wars. In the First World War, many countries, including the United Kingdom, executed soldiers who demonstrated cowardice or deserted; by the Second World War, countries such as the UK and the USA recognized that these behaviours were not necessarily cowardice but traumatic stress – battle shock or combat fatigue had taken over from shellshock – and that troops needed to be treated rather than court-martialled. In Germany and Russia, they were still shot.

A lot of research into traumatic stress was carried out during and after the war, but this was quickly forgotten until the USA became involved in the Vietnam War in the 1960s. Many troops returned home from Vietnam with serious psychological problems, and it was research into these problems that led directly to the introduction of the construct of PTSD in 1980: PTSD was originally concerned with war trauma. Since then, the construct has developed and changed, and it is now used for a range of symptoms, which are discussed in later chapters.

It is important to note at this stage that most people do not develop problems after experiencing a traumatic event. It is only a minority who develop significant clinical symptoms. Many people do have temporary distress, which is not surprising considering that a traumatic event is by definition life-threatening, and therefore frightening.

Defining PTSD

It is not easy to classify traumatic stress. PTSD is only part of the array of reactions experienced by people who go through traumatic experiences. Most people with PTSD are also classified with accompanying – or 'comorbid' – disorders such as depression, generalized anxiety, substance abuse or social disorders. This does create difficulties for terminology, so here, unless otherwise specified, we will use 'traumatic stress' and 'PTSD' interchangeably as both describe what happens to people who are traumatized.

The structure of the book

The book covers the range of problems and issues relating to PTSD and trauma. It does not provide an alternative to therapy for those with PTSD, but it will help develop an understanding of the disorder, and hopefully provide a few tips for helping you come to terms with your problems. The book is also designed to be helpful for relatives and friends trying to understand what a traumatized loved one is going through.

The next chapter focuses on what we mean by a traumatic event. It is important to differentiate between a traumatic event and a stressful event – the term 'stress' is somewhat overused and can be confusing. Although we often use the same coping strategies for general everyday stress as well as traumatic stress, it is important to understand the differences, so we will explore these differences and provide examples of different kinds of stressful and traumatic events.

Chapter 3 focuses on the symptoms of traumatic stress. We have already discussed some of these, and noted how the construct of PTSD does not really cover the range of symptoms people often experience, so Chapter 3 will look at all the key symptoms of PTSD, such as intrusive recollections (the strong emotional memories associated with the traumatic event), avoidance and emotional numbing, and hyperarousal, along with accompanying disorders such as depression and anxiety, substance abuse and social problems, which are common for someone who is traumatized but not necessarily present in everyone diagnosed with PTSD.

Chapter 4 focuses on the key problem associated with traumatic stress, the traumatic memory. All the symptoms of trauma revolve around the traumatic memory, which is a memory that is out of conscious control and that may emerge into consciousness at any time, particularly when the person is reminded of the traumatic event. The traumatic memory may involve cognitive, emotional and even behavioural elements, and the person may not be able to think of the event without the flood of emotions associated with that event. Chapter 4 explores what psychologists know about the traumatic memory, from biological to cognitive and social explanations.

Chapter 5 looks at coping and appraisal. We all cope with problems in different ways, but there are common patterns. When talking about traumatic stress we find that most people tend to be either 'avoiders', who do not like to be reminded of the event, or 'processors', who try to think through the event and make sense of it. In reality, most of us use both strategies at different times – just as we do for normal stressors. It is not just what happened that is important regarding traumatic stress, but the way we think about it, our appraisal of it. Also, one of the key elements regarding recovery from trauma is social support: this means different things to each of us but, as humans, most of us want some kind of human support to help us through our difficult experiences.

Chapter 6 looks at the various ways we tell stories of the traumatic event. We are all storytellers: we have stories about all aspects of our lives and we tell these to other people. The life story we tell our closest friend may not be the same as that we tell our work colleagues, but each is important. Telling the story of the traumatic event is also important. In some ways, an event is only traumatic because we cannot tell it as a story; and we cannot tell it as a story because it does not make sense to us. The purpose of therapy is to help you make sense of the traumatic event, to help you think of it as a narrative or story. This obviously links to social support, as every story needs an audience. It is also linked to the social world, because the way we tell stories, and their content, depends on the social constructs given to us by the world around us, the media, our friends.

Chapter 7 is concerned with how we treat PTSD. It looks at a range of different treatments, but focuses mainly on cognitive behavioural therapy (CBT) and on narrative techniques while briefly exploring other methods such as eye movement desensitization and reprocessing (EMDR), drug treatments and psychoanalysis. All these methods are linked by the narrative, the story.

Chapter 8 focuses on the issues to be dealt with by those living with or caring for the traumatized person. It can often be very difficult for loved ones, particularly if the person with PTSD is socially and emotionally withdrawn or aggressive, as in the cases of Jason and Kate outlined at the beginning of this chapter. It may be hard to understand why someone gets angry or is not as loving as usual. As we have seen, PTSD may appear slowly over years, so it can be difficult to show that, for example, it is caused by a war that finished years previously. Both the person with PTSD and his or her loved ones need to work together to deal with traumatic stress. Chapter 8 also examines secondary trauma, which is where someone who listens to another person's story may in turn be affected by it. This may be the person's family or friends, or therapists or aid workers in war situations. This is not to say that trauma can actually be transmitted, but those who deal a lot with traumatized people may experience problems relating to the stories they hear. This goes back to the narrative or story. Most stories need an audience, so if family members are the audience for a narrative relating to a traumatic event, it can be difficult for them too.

Chapter 9 is concerned with the way many people experience psychological growth because of their traumatic event. It may be that they are initially traumatized but, by working it through, their philosophy of life changes and they realize that they have grown as a person as a result of the traumatic event. They may have learned something about the value of life and death or the meaning of love, or have changed the way they think about how one should live life.

Chapter 10 looks at the professional help that is available for traumatized people, from general practitioners (GPs) and clinical psychologists through to psychiatrists and other therapists. There is a range of mental-health workers and a variety of charities that provide help for individuals suffering from PTSD and related disorders and their families, and at the end of the book we provide details of how to contact such groups.

Chapter 11 brings together the material in the book and draws conclusions. This book will not provide all the answers. It does not serve as an alternative to therapy for seriously affected people, but we hope that it will help people gain some understanding both of themselves and of the processes that are involved in traumatic stress.

At the end of the book is an Appendix that provides a series of self-report measures that you can complete and so gain a little more understanding of your problem. These measures are not an alternative to a full assessment by a therapist, but they may, if completed honestly, give you some indication of the extent of your symptoms. The Further reading section lists a range of books, plays, films and poetry that has described trauma in all its facets. This is not a comprehensive list, but it does serve to indicate the narrative nature of trauma, and contains some of our favourite examples.

2

What is a traumatic event?

Geoff and Sandy
Geoff and Sandy were driving home from a restaurant one evening
when they had an accident. While they were not seriously hurt physically, the driver of the other car suffered severe but not life-threatening
head injuries and numerous broken bones. He did make a full recovery.
Both Geoff and Sandy said afterwards that they thought they were
going to die, and they had moments of utter terror until they realized the accident was over and they were alive. It was not clear who
was to blame for the accident, and in the end the decision was made
that one of the drivers – it was not certain who – had momentarily lost
control. Blame was thus shared, and the insurance companies paid out
accordingly.

Sandy had been driving at the time, and fortunately she had no
serious problems, quickly managing to put the experience behind her,
but Geoff did experience the symptoms of PTSD: nightmares, a sense of
guilt for the accident (he was not driving because he had been drinking
at the restaurant) and anxiety. These symptoms persisted for some time
and had some serious consequences, as we shall see.

The initial research into PTSD focused on war experience as the
traumatic experience. Research in the last 30 years, along with
continuing research on the effects of war, has extended the
concept to include rape, sexual abuse, natural and manmade
disasters, road traffic accidents, and sometimes the death of a
significant other. The nature of the traumatic event, and the
differences between such events and 'normal' events, will be
considered in this chapter.

The classification systems used for mental disorders, the
Diagnostic and Statistical Manual of Mental Disorders (DSM,
published by the American Psychiatric Association), and the
International Classification of Diseases (ICD, published by the

World Health Organization), both accept PTSD as a valid diagnostic concept, and both first introduced PTSD around the same time. Both systems require a series of diagnostic criteria that collectively form a syndrome. For PTSD, one of these diagnostic criteria is the traumatic event itself. There has always been some confusion about the definition of a traumatic event. The initial research leading to the introduction of PTSD was nearly all concerned with war-related events, specifically the US experience in Vietnam in the 1960s and 1970s. Of course, war is a complex experience encompassing many different kinds of event, from killing to being shelled, from rape to seeing one's friends being blown to pieces; but war is not unique in providing the environment for a traumatic response.

A person cannot be diagnosed with PTSD without having experienced a traumatic event. This makes the event itself central to the diagnosis, which is unusual for a mental disorder as most disorders focus on the symptoms themselves rather than what has caused them. The traumatic event is still the first criterion, Criterion A, in *DSM*.

The changing definition of the traumatic event

When PTSD was first brought into the 1980 edition of *DSM* (known as *DSM-III*), the traumatic event was seen as a catastrophic event outside the range of normal human experience. This early definition of the traumatic event criterion seems at one level to be a good definition; it was intended to include major catastrophic events such as war, rape and genocide, natural disasters such as earthquakes and volcanic eruptions, and man-made disasters such as aeroplane crashes and car accidents. There is an assumption that the person has, by being exposed to the above, experienced a very real threat to life. The problem arose that, by using the notion of 'outside the range of normal human experience', the definition ended up excluding things that were commonly experienced, such as the death of a loved one – and logically (by using the concept of 'normal') it failed to recognize that war experience has been, and still is, very common for many millions of people across the world.

DSM-III was trying to distinguish between a traumatic stressor and the normal stressors of everyday life, such as stress associated with work or family. It was assumed that people could cope more effectively with the latter (and if they could not, then they had an adjustment disorder rather than PTSD); this distinction between a traumatic stressor and a 'normal' stressor has been debated ever since.

This can be illustrated by Geoff and Sandy's case, above. Both had the same experience (though Sandy was driving): they were both threatened with death or serious injury, both experienced fear and horror during and immediately after the event, but only Geoff experienced symptoms of PTSD later. While it could be argued that Geoff's PTSD relates to his feelings of guilt that he should have been driving, the reality of the life-threatening experience was the same for both people. Nevertheless, this does show that Geoff's interpretation of what happened (his appraisal) is important in determining whether symptoms will be experienced.

The definition of the traumatic stressor was changed for the 1987 edition of *DSM* and again for the 1994 edition, and is now more open about what the traumatic stressor can be. The criterion is in two parts. The first part is that a person has been exposed to a catastrophic event that involved actual or threatened death or injury, or a threat to the physical integrity of the person or other people. The second part is that the person's reaction, his or her subjective response, involved intense fear, horror or helplessness. This does seem to fit Geoff and Sandy's case, regarding both the threat and the interpretation.

The new definition has proved more useful, as it does not constrain the definition of traumatic stressor and focuses instead on the response of the individual, rather than the event itself. As we shall see in later chapters, PTSD is not just about the event that is experienced. People are so different that we cannot predict who will get PTSD on the basis of an event; it is much more to do with coping skills and appraisal of the event. If 100 people experience a particular event, perhaps only 10 to 20 may be traumatized. The rest may cope very well, as we shall explore in Chapter 5.

Stress and traumatic stress

One area of disagreement among researchers and clinicians is deciding whether a traumatic stressful event is really any different from other stressful events. As we shall see, the coping strategies that people use are common across all stressful events, so it may not be worth making that differentiation. Some people do argue that Criterion A, the traumatic stressor, should be taken out of the definition of PTSD because it is so vague as to be meaningless. If we are talking about a threat to one's life then that threat is not necessarily objective; it is about how we interpret an event. What I see as an actual threat to my life you may not see in the same way. How one person responds to the unexpected death of a loved one is different from how others respond. There are millions of soldiers who have been through terrible events, but only a minority of them go on to develop PTSD. For these reasons, people argue that Criterion A should be abolished because it is too difficult to define.

On the other hand, there is evidence that the kinds of reactions some people have after a catastrophic event are very different from those experienced under normal stress. The symptoms, which we shall look at in detail in the next chapter, can be very much more serious, as they can involve a complete breakdown of normal functioning. With traumatic stress, a person's views about the world can be completely broken down; he or she does not trust people any more and may have ceased to believe in the world as a good place, populated by good people. On the other hand, people who are having problems with the normal stress of work and life may experience a sense of mental exhaustion, but they do not lose faith in the world in the same way as a traumatized person. A person who experiences stress at work or in the family may have depression, but does not have the fundamental destruction of beliefs that can occur as a result of a traumatic experience. The depression in trauma is a secondary result of the event, not a primary response, as it may be in 'normal' stress.

The difficulty, then, is deciding the kinds of events that may lead to a traumatic stress reaction rather than a normal stress reaction. As already noted, it is not possible to provide a comprehensive list, which is why the Criterion A of *DSM* is relatively – and rightly – vague.

Realizing there has been a traumatic event

John

John returned from Afghanistan quite happy. He had served his country, and was proud of how he had performed. He left the army cheerfully, ready to move into civilian life. He did not really have any problems with his memories of what had happened in Afghanistan, though he had experienced some difficult times, particularly when one of his friends from the same platoon was killed by a roadside bomb. He had also helped to clear up the aftermath of a suicide bomb attack, which had killed and injured many civilians. He did not talk about these events to anyone, and everyone thought that there were no problems. It was not until some time later that John began to dwell on these memories and that they started to trouble him. He would be woken in the middle of the night thinking about his friend, or thinking about the sights and smells of the bombing.

This shows the potential difficulty of pinpointing the traumatic stressor. It may not even be prominent in a person's memory for some time after an event. Not only would a clinician fail to notice the memory of the traumatic event, but neither too would the person him- or herself. This makes it very complicated, as the event is not traumatic until the person has the traumatic memory of that event, and this may not occur until months or years after the event took place.

What counts as a traumatic event?

We shall see in the next chapter the range of symptoms that occur in someone who experiences traumatic events. What is not clear is exactly how to define a traumatic event, to provide a list of events that can be traumatic and ones that cannot be traumatic. While it is clear that experiencing war or rape can be traumatic, should we include events such as witnessing an event such as the Hillsborough football disaster on television? There are examples listing the events that people have described as traumatic, but none of these is definitive. For our purposes, we can assume that if a person believes an event to be traumatic, then it is.

3

What are the symptoms?

Pete

Pete had served with the paratroopers in the Falklands War in 1982. He had been involved in a battle where he was caught in crossfire in a trench on the side of a hill. He was trapped in the trench for an hour, and then, as the enemy were pushed back, he advanced again, only to be seriously wounded. He was shipped back to the UK and was in hospital for many months being treated for his wounds. While he was there the troops returned to a heroic welcome, and he felt bitter that he had missed out on it. The nurses brought him presents, but he had wanted to be there at the homecoming and he felt forgotten. He was invalided out of the forces as a result of his wounds, and returned home to live with his parents. He was only 21 and had no family of his own. Over the next few years he drifted in and out of several jobs, usually being sacked for being violent, and managed to have several relationships with girls, which usually ended because he either was violent or threatened to be. Throughout this time Pete was angry – angry with himself for getting wounded, angry with the Paratroop Regiment for (as he saw it) chucking him out, angry with his family and friends, and angry with his employers. He also had regular nightmares about being trapped in the trench, where he continually saw his comrades being killed trying to save him (this was not part of reality, it was just the dream). Pete drank too much and got into fights. Eventually, most people avoided him.

Pete had classic symptoms of traumatic stress. He felt guilt and anger, he had intrusive thoughts (his nightmare), he found it difficult dealing with people and holding down a job.

PTSD has only been in *DSM* since 1980, but in the years since then a great deal of research has established it as an important syndrome. Over 20,000 academic articles have been published, and many hundreds of books. A range of symptoms of PTSD have been identified, from memory problems to issues relating to avoidance and denial, emotional numbing, hyperarousal and coping difficulties, alongside many symptoms that do not fall under the construct of PTSD, which is usually comorbid with other disorders such as depression and substance abuse. These are discussed here along with the symptoms of PTSD. The full pattern should always be considered when examining a person's symptoms. These are cognitive, behavioural and emotional. They are interrelated, and when someone is assessed for PTSD they are all taken into consideration.

What is PTSD?

We have already looked at the historical background of the disorder. It entered *DSM* in 1980 and *ICD* in 1979. The description of PTSD is very similar in both. As discussed in the last chapter, it has been revised several times since 1980, drawing on the wealth of research in the area. The last significant changes were made for the fourth edition of *DSM* in 1994.

When looking at the description of PTSD we should remember that this is a medical classification, although many people dispute whether we should have a medical classification system for the problems relating to traumatic stress, because of the complexity and because there is not a straightforward set of symptoms that come together to form a syndrome. We will return to this later. The advantage of using the term 'PTSD' is that it provides not only a useful set of diagnostic criteria that are helpful to the clinician, but also gives the diagnosis a legal basis. If someone is shown to have PTSD that was derived from someone else's negligence, then a legal compensation claim can be made. (The issue of compensation for PTSD is a legal mine-field, and there is a danger of both over- and under-diagnosing the condition because it is so difficult to define; more on this in Chapter 11.)

In order for someone to be classified as having PTSD, there must be:

1 a traumatic event
2 intrusive re-experiencing
3 avoidance and general numbing
4 hyperarousal
5 problems stemming from these symptoms at work and at home
6 a minimum duration of one month.

The traumatic event

As we discussed in detail in Chapter 2, an event (the traumatic event) must have occurred that led to death or serious injury, or the threat of death or serious injury, to either oneself or others. This event must also have caused intense fear, helplessness or horror. We have seen that the kinds of events that are often considered to be traumatic range from war to rape, natural and manmade disasters, car accidents and assault on the person.

Intrusive re-experiencing

You must have intense uncontrollable memories of the event. These memories may emerge into consciousness at different times, usually cued by some reminder; they may be flashbacks, where you think you are back at the time of the event, or they may be recurring nightmares. The traumatic memory is central to traumatic stress, and we will look at it in more detail in the next chapter, when we look at theoretical aspects of trauma. Briefly, a traumatic memory has cognitive, emotional and behavioural components. What is thought to happen when you are traumatized is that you form an immediate memory of how you felt and behaved at the time. It is instantly imprinted into memory in a very strong indelible form. Why this occurs is not certain, but it is thought that the memory is particularly strong because, if the person behaved in a certain way in a life-threatening situation and survived, then in the future, faced with the same threat, he or she could respond instantly in the same way. The behaviour that proved a life-saver in the first situation might serve the same function a second time. So the traumatic memory can be a good survival mechanism, an adaptive response to the situation. Unfortunately, something that is adaptive in a dangerous life-threatening situation may not be adaptive in everyday situations.

The traumatic memory is often brought into consciousness by a reminder. This can be something directly related to the event, such as a war film for a veteran or going near the place of the rape for a rape victim, or it may be indirect, something in the environment that may not even be recognized as a cue, such as a smell or a sound. Once the memory is activated, there may be cognitive, affective and possibly behavioural consequences. The cognitive component is concerned with going over in the mind what actually happened, and repeating the beliefs associated with the memory (e.g. 'I should have behaved differently', 'My friend might have survived if I had been there', 'I feel guilty that I survived when so many others died'). These memories tend to be detailed, and are usually repeated over and over again, often in exactly the same way. The affective or emotional component is frequently the most difficult part, because it is a reliving of the fear and horror of the time, a re-experiencing of the same feelings again and again. The behavioural component does not always occur, but when it does it can be the most difficult part, especially for the people around the traumatized person: this is when the person may become argumentative and violent, or re-enacts something that happened during the traumatic event.

It is often the case that a traumatic memory does not include all three components. A person may become violent without understanding why this is happening. There may be no obvious relationship between the traumatic event and the later aggression and violence. This again can be very damaging for families, because the family may feel that they are somehow at fault – otherwise, why would the person with PTSD be getting violent?

Nightmares can be very difficult to deal with. Recurrent frightening nightmares may make people feel that they do not want to go to sleep because they are afraid. One war veteran wakes up every night after the same nightmare. He has to get out of bed and change his pyjamas, while his wife changes the bed sheets. Everything is soaked with sweat.

Avoidance and emotional numbing

The traumatic recollections are so painful that you may avoid situations that remind you of the event, and try not to think about what happened. You may use alcohol or other drugs to help you forget. You may also experience difficulties with expressing emotion – not only the negative emotions associated with the event, but also the positive emotions, love, joy or happiness. This can have a serious effect on your relationships. These two interrelated reactions are very common in PTSD. A person who wants to avoid remembering the traumatic event will use any means to avoid reminders, whether these reminders involve not visiting a certain place, not seeing particular people or refusing to talk about what happened. The use of alcohol or other drugs as a means of forgetting can be dangerous if taken to extremes: drugs can lead to dependence and many other problems, and the over-dependence on such supports can harm relationships.

Emotional numbing is a form of avoidance as it involves suppressing (consciously or unconsciously) all emotions. If a person suppresses the positive emotions associated with life then this may lead to problems with relationships – and social support is very important as a means of dealing with the symptoms of traumatic stress.

If you are traumatized you may go through cycles of having intrusive thoughts followed by avoidance, then thoughts may intrude again, and so on. It is a means by which you learn to cope with your memories. A period of intrusive recollecting helps you process the traumatic information, to come to terms with it. However, this is also emotionally draining, so you may then turn to avoidance as a means of coping, in order to have a rest from the burden of memory.

Hyperarousal

You have physiological symptoms associated with the event. These might be problems with concentrating on and attending to tasks, difficulty getting to sleep or staying asleep, or being edgy or easily startled. These are common symptoms, and related to intrusive recollections. If you are constantly thinking about and worrying about your memory of the event then it is likely you will not be able to sleep, you may be startled when you are reminded of the event or, because you feel emotionally drained, you may simply be unable to focus for long on whatever tasks you have to do.

Problems at work and at home

The above symptoms, for a classification of PTSD, must also create problems with work, family or social life. It is not difficult to see that if you are experiencing intrusive thoughts, avoidance and hyperarousal you are likely to have difficulties both at work and at home. If you are unable to concentrate on your job you will not be effective in your work, and this could lead to your being sacked; at home, if you are distracted, emotionally drained or unable to communicate properly then this may lead to significant problems with your partner and family. All these things can exacerbate the situation, as the worse things get at home or work, the worse the symptoms are likely to be.

A minimum duration of one month

The symptoms described above must be experienced for a minimum of one month to be given a diagnosis of PTSD. If the symptoms last for more than three months it is classified as chronic PTSD. If the symptoms do not appear until at least six months after the event it is classified as delayed-onset PTSD. In reality, these figures are somewhat arbitrary. It is not uncommon for someone to have delayed-onset PTSD where the PTSD has developed decades after the traumatic experience, nor is it uncommon for someone to experience PTSD for many years if it is not dealt with effectively.

What other symptoms and disorders are people likely to experience?

People with PTSD usually have comorbid disorders, other symptoms associated with the traumatic event. As we have seen, this can create problems with the definition of PTSD in medical terms, as most medical disorders are discrete sets of symptoms which come together systematically to form a specific disorder. This rarely happens with PTSD. Most people with PTSD are also diagnosed with another disorder. The most common co-disorder is depression, though substance abuse, often using alcohol, is also very common.

Depression

People with PTSD often experience depression. Depression is not just about sadness or being in a low mood; it is far more serious, and it can be difficult to recover, depending on the type of depression. To be classified as depressed, someone must be in a depressed mood nearly every day, with a diminished interest in most normal activities, may possibly have problems with weight gain or loss, sleep, fatigue and concentrating on tasks, and may possibly have suicidal thoughts. These symptoms must seriously affect the person's working or social life, and must not be the direct effects of, for example, the abuse of drugs or medication. For full details of the symptoms, see the checklist in the Appendix.

One study showed that 99 per cent of a sample of war veterans with PTSD also experienced depression, so if you are feeling upset about your traumatic event then do not be surprised that it also makes you depressed. Traumatized people, because they have social difficulties arising from their symptoms and perhaps because their memories not only traumatize them but also make them unhappy, often feel depressed. Owing to the nature of trauma, there is a deep sense of loss – often because a loved one has been killed, though sometimes because of the loss of a sense that the world is a safe and secure place, and the feeling that there is danger lurking around every corner. Sometimes, a person needs to be treated for depression as much as for PTSD. Sometimes the treatment can be psychological; sometimes it is important to have drug treatment.

Anxiety

PTSD is – at least in part – a form of anxiety, and if you have PTSD you may experience anxiety that generalizes outside of the specific traumatic event, making you feel anxious for much of the time, even when you are not thinking about the traumatic event. Again, this is very common. The symptoms of generalized anxiety include a sense of being fearful and tense, and there may be associated physical symptoms such as an increased heart rate, palpitations, shaking, sweating, feeling sick, having a dry mouth, headaches and uncontrolled breathing. Many of the symptoms are linked to PTSD, as they also include an inability to concentrate, feeling edgy or not being able to sleep properly. Remember that anxiety is normal in many circumstances: we all feel these symptoms. A problem arises only when these symptoms are experienced on a regular, perhaps daily, basis. For a full symptom checklist, please see the Appendix.

Substance abuse

This is often taken to mean drinking too much alcohol, too often, but it also refers to the use of illegal drugs such as cocaine, heroin, LSD, amphetamines or cannabis. Many of us turn to alcohol when we are upset, and there is no real problem with having a drink (or several) to help you cope. However, things are different when having a drink becomes a continual habit and you can only deal with your life when you are having a drink. To paraphrase Evelyn Waugh, it is acceptable to drink to get drunk, but not to drink to forget everything that is bothering you.

The problem is that substance abuse does not appear over-night; it is usually a gradual increase in the amount of drinking (or drug-taking) that you and others around you may not notice until it has become a significant issue. Once it becomes a problem for you, it is also a problem for those around you, whether this is because you start to treat people badly, fail to do your work well or spend too much money. In many cases, it can end with physical illness and hospitalization, prison or divorce, and can lead to many health problems such as heart and liver disease.

The symptoms of substance abuse include a number of issues. Again, many of these are related to PTSD, and it is not a simple matter to differentiate PTSD and these comorbid disorders. The symptoms include: giving up past activities such as hobbies and sports; doing less well at work; aggression; forgetfulness; depression; lack of money; being selfish; using room deodor-izers to remove smells; getting drunk or high on a regular basis; lying about the use of alcohol or drugs; hangovers; encouraging others to drink or use drugs; getting into legal problems; drink-driving; indulging in risky behaviour; blackouts. Again, there is a symptom checklist in the Appendix.

Effects on others

The above shows why the response to traumatic stress is very complicated. It is not just about a set of symptoms or diagnostic criteria that relate to PTSD, it is the range of other symptoms that you might experience; and because these – including PTSD – have such an effect not only on you yourself but also on the people around you, they may become even more complicated as time progresses. If a person reacts to your symptoms of depression or anger, then you may react to him or her. If someone gets angry because you are angry, then the cycle of violence may increase. If you upset your wife or husband because you are constantly depressed, then you are likely to feel worse rather than better. It is unfortunately too common that serious rifts result from people being unable to cope with a loved one's behaviour, and this can be dangerous, particularly for war veterans, because of the resultant aggression and violence. For this reason it is important that any treatment or help you receive takes into account the social side of traumatic stress, and your relationships with family and friends.

Self-assessment

If you wish, you can complete the self-report measures in the Appendix to find out more about your own symptoms. This will provide a rough indication of whether you may or may not have PTSD. A diagnosis of the disorder (and of the other disorders listed in the Appendix which have checklists) can only be made by a properly qualified person, so please do not take a high score to indicate that you have PTSD, only that you might need further help and advice and that you should seek help from a qualified person. You can obtain access to professional help via your GP (see Chapter 10 for further details).

Bearing in mind that these measures are not a substitute for a clinical diagnosis by a qualified professional, the self-report measures – completed honestly – will provide you with a basic account of what you are facing. With this information, you can start to work out how you can get better.

4

What are traumatic memories?

John, the veteran of the Afghan War we met in Chapter 2, experienced serious problems with his traumatic memories. He had terrible dreams that woke him up, all relating to his experiences in Afghanistan. When he woke he could not tell whether he was asleep or awake, whether he was in Afghanistan or England. The fear and horror of his memories flooded back to him, uncontrollably, so that he would sometimes weep.

Jim, a veteran of the Second World War, a paratrooper who jumped 42 times including in Normandy and across the Rhine, would describe his traumatic experiences of battle. The descriptions were very vivid and detailed, and sometimes I would wonder how he remembered so much. Then I saw his living room, and it was packed with books and videos about the war. Jim's memories were amalgamations of what had really happened to him, and what he had later read about or seen. That is not to say his memories were not truthful, just that over time he had incorporated more details into them to make sense of the fighting he witnessed and took part in. He de-traumatized his memories by making sense of them, in a way we will describe in Chapter 6.

Traumatic memories are central to our understanding of the response to traumatic events. They differ from normal memories in being out of control and in being associated with emotional and behaviour components, as well as cognitive elements. In order to understand trauma and memory, it is important to understand the different perspectives psychology uses to build theory, from socio-cultural explanations to the underlying biology, the brain mechanisms that are affected in PTSD and comorbid disorders. An evolutionary approach will help us understand how and why people respond to stressors in the ways they do.

Memory

Memories are complex. In the past, many psychologists have studied them as though they were stored versions of reality, with a simple relationship between input (information from the outside world), storage (keeping this information in the brain in some way) and output (recalling the information). They also assumed that the recalled information tended to be accurate, though perhaps subject to decay ('I cannot recall everything about the event') or interference ('I get my memories mixed up'). This is a gross oversimplification of the way memory works. In the 1970s people started to think about different types of memories: for instance, the difference between the memories of things that have happened to us (e.g. 'What did I have for breakfast today?') and things that we can do, such as riding a bike or driving a car. Memories such as riding a bike involve something we cannot fully describe but can do, i.e. it is nonverbal, implicit and somehow non-conscious. Memories for things that have happened can be described, such as eating smoked fish and salad for breakfast; these memories are verbal, explicit and conscious. We will return to this distinction later, as it is important for understanding traumatic memory.

Francis Bartlett, writing in the 1930s, understood a lot about memory. Unfortunately his work was largely ignored by many psychologists until relatively recently. Bartlett understood that memory was not about simply remembering facts, events and how to do things. We do not remember exactly what happened: we interpret events and remember that interpretation. This memory may then change over time as a result of re-interpretation, experience, or motivation – for instance, there are aspects of our lives we may choose not to remember because they are embarrassing or unpleasant. We actively remember the most important events and forget those that are less important. We make sense of things that happen to us, and the process of making sense affects what is remembered and how it is remembered.

The concept of narrative memory has relevance here, in the sense that narrative is about the ways in which we tell our life stories. Narrative is explored more thoroughly in Chapter 6, which discusses the telling of the story of the traumatic event, but narrative also has a major impact on memory. A narrative is a story that we tell others (or sometimes tell ourselves) about some aspect of our lives. Clearly, depending on the audience, we will focus more strongly on certain aspects of our lives, certain memories, than on others; and the story itself will depend on the audience. One is likely to say certain things to friends and relations that one would not say to strangers or work colleagues. How we develop and use these narratives depends on many circumstances, both personal and social. This will affect how we draw on our memories, which ones we discuss or discard, how we manipulate and change them. While some might argue this is a form of misrepresenting the truth, because we deliberately over- or under-emphasize aspects of our lives, it is what we all do, both consciously and unconsciously; it is a perfectly normal human process, and within the context of traumatic stress it is a very useful human process.

These effects occur in all aspects of life, which is why two people who have the same experience will remember it differently. How it is remembered may depend on someone's mood at the time, how important it is perceived to be and whether it is a unique event or something out of the ordinary. As we shall see, this has clear implications for traumatic memory.

The other important distinction between types of memory is that between short-term temporary memory and long-term permanent memory. Short-term or working memory refers to the information that is held in the head consciously, e.g. when you are trying to remember a phone number or address, or when you are thinking about what someone is saying to you.

Long-term memory is the information that is stored in a more or less permanent manner in the brain.

It is important to understand something of the way in which ordinary memory works in order to understand traumatic memory, which makes use of the same basic processes but in a dysfunctional way.

Traumatic memory

Traumatic memories are memories of terrible, frightening, horrific events where the person cannot control the memory, which is associated with fear, helplessness or horror. Traumatic memories tend to be very vivid, not just visually but also for sound and often for smell. They emerge into consciousness unpredictably, day and night, and the person typically tries to control them by avoiding reminders of the event, by staying clear of the place the event happened or the people who also took part, or by not watching reminders on the television. Often, these memories are not effectively controlled in this way, and when a traumatic memory is recalled it is associated not only with the cognitive elements but also with the emotions and feelings associated with the event, and sometimes with behaviour too. A further problem with traumatic memories is that, when they become conscious, the fear and horror associated with them can exacerbate the situation by strengthening that link between the memory and the emotion. If we want to make people better, then that link needs to be broken. We will be discussing ways of doing this in later chapters.

> Dave was in an infantry unit in Iraq, going out on regular patrols in the difficult times of 2006. Dave had many difficult and frightening experiences, and was particularly upset by the consequences of a roadside bomb that exploded near his patrol. He was walking near his good friend when the bomb went off. A piece of metal sliced off the top of his friend's skull, leaving him dying in the road. Many people were killed and injured, but Dave went to his friend and saw the emotions in his

eyes – everything from calmness to fear – as he died. The image that Dave finds difficult is seeing his friend's eyes moving and at the same time seeing the top of his brain. He was oblivious to what was happening around him.

When Dave returned to the UK, he didn't really talk about his experiences, apart from a very general way. The other things that had happened didn't really bother him too much, even though some were quite horrific: it was the single image of his friend's eyes and brain that wouldn't go away. This was the traumatic memory. Dave thought of it night and day. It came into his dreams, and it confronted him in his garden. There was no peace. And it was always the same, never-changing image.

When we discuss PTSD we think of fear, horror and helplessness. For Dave, it was the horror and helplessness that dominated. He hadn't been able to help his friend, and he felt guilty that he survived and his friend didn't. And what made it much worse was that he knew his friend's wife really well, and he couldn't tell her how he died.

Understanding traumatic memories

Traumatic memories make more sense if we understand something about the processes involved in such memories. As we have already discussed, traumatic memories are related to ordinary memory processes; indeed, what we want to happen is for a traumatic memory to be turned into an ordinary memory. Pierre Janet, a French clinician who worked towards the end of the nineteenth and into the early twentieth centuries and who focused an important part of his work on trauma, made a simple but accurate observation. He suggested that the role of therapy in trauma is to turn the traumatic memory into a narrative memory, i.e. to make sense of the traumatic event so that it can be incorporated into the person's life story (we will discuss this at length in Chapter 6). The principle applies to all forms of therapy for traumatic stress: we are always trying to turn the traumatic memory into the narrative memory.

First of all, we need to explore the nature of traumatic memories.

Theoretical aspects of traumatic memories

As already noted, there are a number of aspects of ordinary memory that play an important role in traumatic memories. While we are not sure of the exact processes, it is thought that traumatic memories are processed differently from ordinary memories. There are several brain pathways via which memories are stored, but two are particularly pertinent in understanding traumatic memory: the hippocampal pathway and the thalamo-amygdala pathway. In simple terms, these are the pathways that are relevant for explicit and implicit memories respectively. The amygdala, the thalamus and the hippocampus are all sub-cortical structures within the brain with complex roles (see Figure 1). Here, we are only referring to them in respect of the part they play in traumatic memory (see Figure 2).

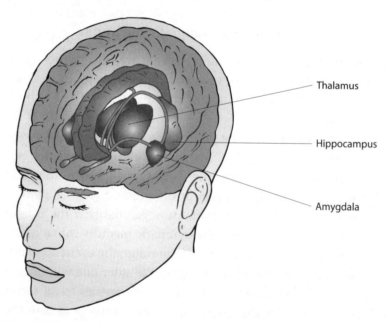

Figure 1 Some key memory structures in the brain

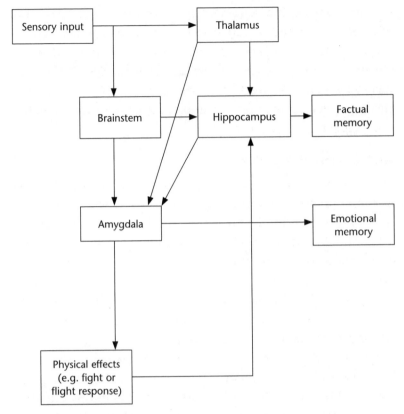

Figure 2 Memory pathways

Hippocampal pathway

The hippocampal pathway is that used for transferring normal memories into long-term memory. It is used for all sorts of memories, from listening to someone describing their garden to remembering where you went for your holidays. It is a conscious, explicit, verbal route, which processes information relatively slowly, with the imprint of a new memory sometimes taking days or weeks to be consolidated. This is also the pathway responsible for enabling us to forget information – forgetting being as important as remembering, for memory. Why would we want to remember what we had for breakfast every day? It is of no relevance (unless you are a chef or food expert, and even then the memory will be lost unless it is recorded in a diary or elsewhere) and so does not clutter up our memories. That is why memories may take weeks to consolidate; it may not become clear whether or not they are important enough to remember until some time after the event.

Thalamo-amygdala pathway

There are many circumstances when the hippocampal pathway is not appropriate for inputting memories, such as when learning a skill that becomes implicit when it is fully learned, such as riding a bike or driving a car. It is not possible to describe verbally exactly how to conduct this type of skill, and in these instances other pathways are used. One of these pathways, which we think is important for traumatic memories, is the thalamo-amygdala pathway. This is a rapid, non-conscious, implicit pathway that allows for very rapid input and storage of information.

This pathway is very useful in a life-threatening situation. If a person's life is threatened, he or she may need to respond very quickly in order to survive. Most responses in this situation are reflexive, automatic. If it is a war situation then a soldier is trained to behave automatically in many situations. These rapid responses are basic survival mechanisms, many of which have evolved to enable an organism to survive longer. The problem with people is that we have complicated the survival mechanism by having complex thoughts, feelings and behaviours. A far greater proportion of our behaviours are learned than is the case for other animals. Also, our cognitive abilities, our intelligence, along with our emotional responses, are more sophisticated. While we normally think these sophisticated responses are what sets us above the animals, in the case of a traumatic life-threatening experience they may often set us below other animals.

During a traumatic event the normal slow hippocampal route is cut off – there is evidence that hippocampal damage is caused by the rush of adrenaline that occurs in a threatening situation – and the very rapid thalamo-amygdala route comes into action, enabling both a rapid response and the rapid imprint of that response into long-term memory. The survival mechanism element is that the rapid imprint of the memory will enable you, if you are faced with the same threat in the future, to respond quickly again, to respond in the same way, which assisted your survival.

To take a crude example, after the Second World War there was a classic tale of how veterans would automatically fall to the ground when a car backfired. They had learned this response both in training and on the battlefield. A soldier who hits the ground when the firing starts is more likely to survive through presenting a smaller target to the enemy. This is a conditioned response, one over which the person has little or no control. It is a good survival mechanism on the battlefield, but it looks very silly, at best, when walking down a street in peacetime.

If we take this example further, the association between the stimulus (car backfiring) and the behavioural response (falling flat on the ground) is automatic, but that is not the only response. There is usually the fear and horror associated with one's life being threatened – the emotional response – and there are the beliefs, the thoughts that one is going to die, that one's friends are going to die. All these responses are activated automatically.

This then is the traumatic memory. It is the cognitive, emotional and behavioural response to a stimulus that activates a terrible memory of a traumatic event. It is out of the control of the person, and it is extremely distressing. It is a very strong and negative memory of the life-threatening event. Clearly, people who have been through complex traumas such as war or child sexual abuse may have many traumatic memories, which can be triggered by many different stimuli.

Traumatic memories can emerge in the daytime during the person's everyday life. There may be no clear reminder: the memory just emerges. The memory may emerge at night when the person is resting, or as a nightmare during sleep. Typically, nightmares are repetitive; typically, all traumatic memories are repetitive. They are known collectively as 'traumatic re-experiencing'.

Limitations to understanding

Our understanding of traumatic memories is reasonably good, but there are many limitations, as will become obvious through the next few chapters. If a group of, say, 100 people experience a particular life-threatening event then, as we have seen in previous chapters, not all of them will develop traumatic memories. Of those that do, the memories will differ between people; they will also differ in terms of time span. Some people will have traumatic memories immediately after an event; others will not experience any such memories at first, but they may develop over the next few months, years or even decades. There is no clear pattern of response and there are no clear patterns of traumatic memories – apart from the fact that they are being extremely intense cognitively, emotionally and sometimes behaviourally.

In the next chapter we shall explore some of these individual differences in the experience of traumatic memories, and show how it is not what a person experiences but how they think about it, how they appraise it, that matters.

5

How do we cope with trauma?

Sandy, who we met in Chapter 2, did not experience any serious symptoms of PTSD after a road accident, though her husband Geoff did. Sandy has a good set of friends who she spends quite a lot of time with. She has known several of them for many years, and they know each other very well. After the accident, she confided in one of these friends, Michelle. When Michelle came round to see her, Sandy described what had happened and how she felt, and Michelle chatted with her for a couple of hours, telling Sandy to phone her if she was ever upset. Sandy did phone Michelle a couple of times, but it was more the thought that she had someone to phone and to talk to that seemed to help most, not actually having to phone. When asked, Sandy said that it was the opportunity to chat about what had happened with her friend that – for her – explains why she didn't have any problems. She also let on that Geoff did not have any close friends with whom he shared such detailed and personal emotional information.

Whether or not you become traumatized by your experiences depends not only on what you have experienced but also how you interpret that experience; it depends on your personality and coping styles, social support, your genes and the ways in which you appraise the traumatic situation. This chapter introduces the key areas of coping, and how this links to whether or not someone will experience trauma. There are a number of coping styles that we habitually use not only in traumatic situations, but also in other stressful situations. This chapter will also look at the role of social support, which is widely recognized as being the key factor in determining outcome.

Individual differences

The area of individual differences is an important one in psychology. It is where we look not at how people as a whole behave in a given situation, but at how they differ. Why is it that if two people are exposed to the same traumatic situation, one may be traumatized and the other may display no symptoms whatsoever? Right at the outset we need to say that becoming traumatized does not mean that you are weaker or more worthless than other people; there is no shame in experiencing trauma, and neither is there shame in not experiencing trauma – it doesn't make you shallow and unfeeling. There is a danger in the modern world that people are somehow expected to be traumatized by particular events. This is a dangerous situation. As we stated at the outset, most people are not traumatized. There are many different ways in which people respond to difficult situations, and the purpose of this chapter is to elucidate some of those differences.

> There was a tragic accident at a school, where two school friends from the same year were killed. The headteacher brought in a number of counsellors who spoke individually to every pupil in the same year as those who had been killed, and to each class of the other years. There was an expectation that many children would be traumatized. What they found was that the children resented the counsellors. They did not want to see them. With a couple of exceptions, the children wanted to deal with the deaths in their own way. Most of the children did not know the dead children, and of those who did most were acquaintances. Later, the headteacher did recognize that he had made a mistake: he should have focused on talking to the close friends of the dead children, but with an open door policy for anyone else who wanted to talk.

We know that people differ in many ways. Apart from the obvious physical differences of size, weight, sex, etc., we differ in personality, intelligence, memory, the way we attend to and perceive the world; we differ in upbringing and genes; and we differ in life experiences. Differences in genes and prior experience have a major impact on the ways in which we respond to what is going on around us, and that includes the ways we respond to traumatic events.

The response to stress

The classic fight or flight syndrome provides a basic explanation of what happens to us when we undergo stress in the environment (as originally described by Walter Cannon in 1929). Our physiological response to stress exists to help us survive a life-threatening situation. We automatically prepare our bodily defences to fight the threat or to run away. When we perceive a threat, our sympathetic nervous system kicks into action with the release of adrenaline and cortisol, which prepare our body for action. The heart rate quickens, which increases blood pressure, increasing the blood flow to the muscles, supplying them with extra energy for action. At the same time the digestive system is slowed down. Once the threat is over the parasympathetic nervous system adjusts the system back to normal levels by a process known as homeostasis. Stress-related symptoms may occur when someone is experiencing chronic environmental stress; the body is continually preparing for action but no action ensues, so the system becomes disrupted.

The response to traumatic stress is basically similar but has a great degree of involvement of the memory and emotions, as described in earlier chapters.

Coping

Coping is concerned with how we deal with everyday life, how we solve problems, how we interact with the world. It is about mastering problems, learning to tolerate them or reducing the effects of stress. Since the days of Sigmund Freud psychologists have developed many different theories of coping. We have long known that people differ in the ways they deal with events in the world; these differences are quite fundamental and they differ in their effectiveness. Some coping strategies work well, some work less well; some work well in some situations, others work well in different situations. Some people use one set of coping strategies effectively, others use different coping strategies effectively. Some theories of coping have listed up to 15 or 20 different coping strategies, and we cannot say with any certainty that some are better than others; it is the ways they are used by particular people in certain circumstances that make them either helpful or unhelpful.

Most of the research into coping over the last half-century or so has focused on the relationship between stress and coping. More recently, there has been a lot of work on traumatic stress and coping, and this has shown that the basic coping mechanisms that are used are similar for both 'ordinary' stress and traumatic stress. One of us (NCH) carried out his PhD research on the problems experienced over the longer term by war veterans. Part of this work involved looking at coping and showed that people tend to cope in two basic ways: cognitive processing and avoidance. We all use both strategies, but we tend to prefer one or the other. The research also showed that social support plays a crucial role: something we will discuss later.

Processing

'Processing' is a general term that refers to actively thinking about and trying to deal with a problem. People who process their traumatic thoughts may go over them continually in their minds, but manage to work through them in order to make sense of them. Working through the thoughts can take many forms, from just sitting and thinking to writing about them or talking through them with a friend or a therapist. All talking therapy in the end is about helping a person work out his or her problems. If a person has traumatic memories, then it may be that there are several problems relating to those memories.

For instance, it may be that the event led the person to feel guilty about surviving when others may have died; or it may seem impossible to separate the emotions from the memory. By talking it over, working it through, the problem becomes easier to deal with.

A classic example of processing is that of a Second World War veteran who, decades after the war, was mostly psychologically well but would occasionally have reminders that led to traumatic thoughts. He said that if this happened – and he could usually understand what had triggered the memory – then he would take a blank sheet of paper and write a poem. Once the poem was complete then the memory did not cause any further problems. This is a very 'clean' example, and it is rare for someone to be so organized in his or her mind as to be able to resolve traumatic memories in this way. It is usually much more difficult, but such activities as writing or creating art do work, helping people to think about their problems and work them out. There are countless cases of people writing stories, biographies, novels, plays or poetry to deal with their traumatic memories (see examples in Further reading, films and plays); there are also many cases where people have turned to art to achieve the same thing. It can be a form of self-therapy, and it can be very effective.

One difficulty with this kind of coping is that it may become stuck. For many people, dealing with a traumatic memory is so difficult they don't know how to handle it, so it goes over and over in their mind and the actual memory and the thoughts and feelings that go with it don't change; the person is ruminating. This is not processing, as there is no change to the memory. If a person ruminates, this can lead to additional reactions such as depression rather than resolution, as the traumatic memory and its consequences are constantly in the mind. This illustrates just how complicated coping can be.

Avoidance

Avoidance is by far the most common coping strategy among people who have been traumatized. Avoidance refers to people steering clear of anything that might remind them of the traumatic event, such as other people who were involved, the site where it took place or any television coverage. In this way, people seek to avoid having the traumatic memories brought back into consciousness. While on one level this may sound like a negative coping strategy, it can be very positive. If a person can succeed in avoiding thinking about the traumatic event, then he or she will succeed in experiencing fewer symptoms.

However, problems can develop if avoidance is used as a strategy. Research carried out with Second World War veterans showed that many successfully used avoidance for decades, but then started to experience the symptoms of traumatic stress after retirement. What seemed to be happening was that these veterans returned from the war, and then managed to avoid their memories by getting married, having children, working and generally living a normal life. It wasn't until after they retired – when they had more time to think – that they started experiencing traumatic symptoms. Many reported that these symptoms were as serious as those they had during and immediately after the war. Many had nightmares and emotional problems. What appears to happen is that if a person avoids thinking about traumatic memories, it is not that the memories disappear; there is a danger that they will re-emerge at any point in later life. Of course, for many people avoidance may be a successful strategy throughout life.

Processing and avoidance

These examples show how complex coping is; and inevitably most of us regularly use both coping strategies. Indeed, there is evidence that we deliberately use both. Mark Creamer carried out research which showed how traumatized people might go through phases of processing and avoidance. People may attempt to deal with their traumatic memories through processing, but over time this becomes too distressing, so they start to use avoidance in order to rest from the difficult emotions they are trying to deal with. Then, when they are able, they again start using processing in order to deal with the traumatic memories. People may go through several cycles of processing and avoidance before they successfully deal with their memories, and this may take years to complete.

Other coping strategies

People use an array of different coping strategies, many of which can be placed in the context of processing and avoidance. Another distinction is made between problem-focused and emotion-focused coping. With the former, a person will actively think about ways in which to deal with the stressful event or memory. The latter refers to those situations that are more difficult to deal with. So someone who is actively processing the traumatic memories may be using a problem-focused strategy.

Coping is traditionally measured using questionnaires, and these show us the different types of coping people use. There are two very popular questionnaires on the market, COPE and the Ways of Coping Questionnaire. The Ways of Coping Questionnaire records eight distinct ways of coping: confrontive, seeking social support, planful problem-solving, self-control, distancing, positive appraisal, accepting responsibility and escape–avoidance. Studies of this questionnaire do not always agree on these eight forms of coping. As you can probably surmise, some of them do overlap. We can see that planful problem-solving is an active processing strategy that will correlate with self-control and positive appraisal, and that successful processing will be associated with accepting responsibility.

COPE is derived theoretically and has 15 different coping strategies. These include active coping, planning, seeking social support, suppression of competing activities, religion, positive interpretation and growth, restraint, resignation–acceptance, focus on and venting of emotions, denial, mental disengagement, behavioural disengagement, alcohol or drug use and humour. Again, the coping strategies listed here overlap, and we can see how they relate to processing and avoidance.

These measures do provide examples of effective coping. The notion of positive interpretation and growth, present in both questionnaires, is particularly helpful. Positive growth is a relatively new idea in psychology: it suggests that if a person experiences trauma, then he or she may, over time, learn from that experience, and develop into a 'better' person in some way, perhaps with a greater understanding of the value of life or family, or a different perspective on death.

Alcohol and drug use is usually seen in a negative light, but the use of alcohol is a very common coping strategy. It does help people forget their troubles, at least for a time,. Instead of focusing on alcohol in purely negative terms, it is worth considering how it has been used for centuries to help people deal with their problems. People who are drinking are more likely to open up and discuss their traumatic memories with others; and through this they may find ways of dealing with these memories. The trouble with alcohol is that it can lead to a number of serious problems. It makes some people violent, both with their families and others. Prolonged overuse of alcohol can make a person unable to work; it can create serious family difficulties and money problems, and in serious cases it can lead to illness and sometimes death. If someone goes through a traumatic experience and has a few nights or weeks of drinking, then there may not be any need for concern. This arises only when, after the trauma, the person's drinking patterns permanently change and lead to inappropriate behaviours.

Religion serves as a coping strategy for many people, who find meaning and support in their beliefs. By talking to God, or explaining the situation or event in terms of God's will, people find solace. For instance, many Iranian veterans of the Iran–Iraq War (1980–8) believe that their war was a just war, a jihad, fought for Allah. No matter what their situation since the war, whether they are in poverty or whether they are crippled, they may still believe that they fought a just war for Allah.

Another very common coping strategy is black humour, regularly used by emergency workers, people in the armed forces, and others. This is where the person makes a joke about the traumatic situation, the accident, the firefight or whatever. While outsiders might think this inappropriate (perhaps even 'politically incorrect'), it is a very effective and useful strategy. The social niceties of the civilian do not apply to people who regularly deal with the threat of death and serious injury to themselves and others.

Social support

Social support has a different heading from coping because it has fundamental differences. The discussion up to now has focused on individual coping styles which, although the use of them may impact on others, stem largely from the individual. Social support is a much broader concept, one that is critically important for people in any culture and one that has become problematic for many in Western cultures through the high degree of individualism that exists, with many people living alone rather than as a family. This may be leading to more stress and trauma than would otherwise be the case, because good social support really does help people come to terms with their experiences. If one is living alone then there may be no one to talk to, and one might then dwell on the traumatic memory, ruminate, and experience a greater degree of depression as well as trauma.

Perceived social support

One of the problems with much of the research into social support is that it has assumed that the number of people one knows indicates the degree of social support experienced. While this may seem to contradict what has just been said, the effectiveness of social support is more about whether a person perceives that he or she has such support. Many people may experience good social support from a single person, while others may have close relationships with several people but do not feel supported. There are many different ways of thinking about how well your friends and close family provide support.

Social support and war

Research on Second World War veterans carried out by one of us (NCH) showed that the veterans had two very different sorts of social support, and the distinction is probably true for many people who have been traumatized. In the first place, veterans would not talk about their traumatic experiences to their wives and families. They saw the home as a protected place, one where the danger and emotions of trauma should not be present. Home was a safe place, and their wives and families supported them in keeping it that way. The second form of support was provided by other veterans, usually at veterans' association meetings. At these meetings the veterans would discuss in detail what had happened during the war, including rehearsing the traumatic elements. Many veterans said they came away from such meetings in tears as they had been remembering their friends who were killed and what they had been through. But they wanted to have these discussions. They felt that talking about the war helped them. It made them very emotional, but was part of the process of dealing with it.

No return to the pre-trauma state

The veterans' association example illustrates one important aspect of coping: its purpose is not to return someone to the pre-traumatic state, not to 'make them better' as one gets better from a cold or a broken leg, but to enable people to deal with their memories, deal with their emotions, in an effective way, and help them to be able to build on these memories and grow.

Conclusion

There are many different forms of coping, and theoreticians have not been able to produce an agreed list of coping strategies. This is largely because different coping strategies overlap to a greater or lesser extent; they are not separate strategies. Also, we all use a range of strategies to deal with stress and trauma. We use different strategies at different times, and combine strategies to make them work more effectively. The next few chapters discuss particular ways of effectively dealing with traumatic memories. The discussion of coping will help inform our understanding of these methods.

6

Telling the story of the trauma

At the heart of any understanding of traumatic stress lies the disrupted narrative, the story that doesn't make sense. For you to recover from traumatic stress you need to turn your experiences into a story, a means of making sense of what happened to you. This story can be told via therapy, by writing it down, by talking to others, by drawing pictures, or simply by thinking it through. Most stories require an audience, so the role of social support is important – though not always necessary. Stories also depend on the culture in which they are created, so we will explore this too in this chapter.

Tricia

Tricia was raped when she was a teenager. At the time she never told anyone about it. It had happened at a party, when a man she had never met before plied her with drinks, started to walk her home and then attacked her in a field. She felt abused and humiliated. Afterwards she walked home, had a shower and went straight to bed. She didn't report what had happened to the police; she didn't tell her parents. Fortunately there were no visible marks so they did not ask any awkward questions. After the attack she stopped going out. She would tell people that it was because she was concentrating on her A levels. She spent a lot of time in her bedroom, avoiding contact with people, males especially but also her close friends, in whom she usually confided all the details of her life. Her friends realized something was wrong, but only gradually, and over time they came to see her less and less because she would not go out. Tricia did not do well in her A levels and got a job working in a shop, simply because it was the first thing that came along. She had become very passive, and would just go along with what her parents suggested, mainly for an easy life.

Tricia did not at first show the usual signs of being traumatized. She did not have nightmares or symptoms such as hyperarousal. Her response to the rape was to withdraw. While the people around her saw that she had changed, this was explained by her excuse that she was studying. No one saw any reason to investigate further, even her parents. When she did not do well at school it was put down to her studying techniques not being particularly effective. It was only when she had been working for a few months that she started to experience psychological problems relating to the rape. It started with a growing anxiety around people, particularly men, which reminded her of the rape. The memory of the attack started to come back more strongly and she would become tearful. At night she was nervous. The anxiety started to affect her job, and her manager noticed. One day the manager asked to see Tricia, and asked what was wrong. At first Tricia said she didn't know, but the manager was perceptive and sensitive and realized there was a genuine problem. She told Tricia to take a week off to try and sort herself out. She said that when things were bothering her she would sit down with a blank piece of paper and write about them, and that helped. Tricia agreed to take the time off, and began to realize that she needed to deal with her situation.

Tricia went home that day and thought about what her manager had said. She sat down in her bedroom at her computer and for the first time really thought about the rape and how it had affected her. She wrote down everything she could about it. It took her a long time, because she tried to write down every detail. She first of all described the rape itself, then her feelings as she remembered them at the time, and her feelings now. She tried to understand why she felt as she did. The task was exhausting and took several hours. At the end of the time she went to bed and fell fast asleep, sleeping better than she had done for some time. The following day she read through what she had written, and started to revise it, adding details, changing parts she thought were not quite right. She was deliberately trying to find an explanation for the way she felt: the way she felt about the attack, her attacker and her own mixed-up emotions and thoughts.

Tricia repeated this exercise each day for the whole week, and found that by the fifth or sixth day she was making very few changes. She also found that she felt much better about herself. She now began to understand why she felt as she did. She realized that she was perfectly justified in being nervous, but that her nervousness should not stop her from interacting with her friends and colleagues. She admitted to herself that she hated her attacker for what he had done to her – not just the rape, but the way it had changed her over the last couple of years – but she felt justified in hating him. She thought about going to the police but decided not to: as there was no evidence relating to the attack there would be little to gain. She was starting to think rationally again, and she felt she could control her feelings. While this writing exercise didn't make everything perfect again, it helped Tricia to start to socialize, and to get her life back.

Examples such as this are common. While such an exercise would not suit everyone, writing down your thoughts and feelings about a traumatic episode can help you feel better. After a war, many soldiers write detailed accounts of their experiences, not necessarily for publication but just to make sense of their actions and the actions of their comrades and enemies. They sometimes let their family and friends read them, but many accounts stay hidden away or may even be destroyed because the person doesn't want anyone else to see them. Remember the Second World War veteran mentioned in Chapter 5: if his war memories were stirred up, he would simply write a poem about the memory and then he would feel all right again.

As we have already discussed, everyone is different and we all have different ways of dealing with our stressful and traumatic experiences. While writing about one's experiences may not suit everyone, it does suit some people. This chapter is for those people.

There are methods of treatment known as narrative methods, which we will discuss in Chapter 7. For the moment, we will just briefly describe one of them, known as narrative exposure therapy (developed by Frank Neuner and his colleagues). This is a technique that has been used with various groups, particularly refugees, and has been shown to be effective. While it does make use of a therapist, it is essentially a method of developing a meaningful story about one's traumatic experiences. Traumatized people are asked to describe the event, along with their thoughts and feelings. Over a period of days, they revise and develop their account until they consider it satisfactory; just as Tricia did about her thoughts and feelings about the rape. The account is written up as a witness statement and signed by the person, with a view that it could be used in a court of law against the perpetrators of the traumatic incident. This technique is used for a dual purpose: people are creating a potentially useful witness document and at the same time addressing their own reactions. It has been shown to be at least as effective as many more sophisticated techniques.

What these examples suggest is that there are a number of ways of telling the trauma story, whether doing it yourself or having another person there to lead you through the process of describing the incident, and your feelings and thoughts about that incident.

The secret of narrative is that we are all storytellers. It is what we do best. Whether we are at work or in the home, we tell stories to people about our experiences and our thoughts. We tell our friends about our past lives, and our partners about our day at work. A key characteristic of stories is that they are manipulable: they can be reconstructed in any way we choose. We are never objective in our telling of a story. It changes according to the audience (e.g. describing your past life to work colleagues may be different from the description you give your children).

The problem with traumatized people is that they do not have the story of the event that caused the trauma. The memories are often fragmented or dissociated; they do not fit together very well. Those who are traumatized do not understand why they have particular feelings relating to the event; they don't understand their thoughts, their attitudes, their beliefs. It is like a jigsaw, where many of the pieces are sitting on the table but the picture can't yet be made out, and some of the pieces are missing. All forms of therapy for trauma are about piecing these memories, feelings and thoughts back together to make a coherent whole, to make sense of the experience, to make a narrative, a story that makes sense to the person. It is not about recreating the life story that a person had before the traumatic incident, but about enabling the traumatic incident to be put in the past, into memory, rather than constantly reliving it.

Another key element of a story is that there is usually an audience. Occasionally a story is meant only for the person creating the story (e.g. the war journals described above), but nearly always we create a narrative for a specific audience, whether that be family, friend, work colleague or someone you chat to in the street. Research shows that people who have the most effective social support are the ones who are least likely to experience serious symptoms after a traumatic experience. The problem is that many people who have a traumatic experience keep themselves away from their family and friends, the very people they should be relying on for support. This is a key element when thinking about narrative: narratives are designed for an audience.

Narrative therapy is becoming increasingly popular, as we shall see, but many people who are traumatized piece the story together themselves. If they are able to communicate well with their friends and family – or perhaps with one particular person with whom they feel confident about discussing the traumatic event – then they are less likely to have symptoms. The act of talking about a traumatic event in itself is often helpful, as it helps the person to start putting the event into perspective.

But not everyone needs a confidante in order to make sense of their experiences. Many people can just sit and think about it; or go for a walk and think about it.

Cultural factors

Another factor that is important is culture. The narratives that we construct do not only depend on how we as individuals want to tell the story and who we want to tell it to: they depend on the culture in which we live. In some cultures it is acceptable to be very emotional with friends and to discuss personal details; in other cultures it is expected that people keep their feelings to themselves. So how you develop and use your narratives depends on the country in which you live, the time in which you live, and perhaps also the social class to which you belong. For instance, after the Second World War it was not deemed appropriate for returning British soldiers to discuss their experiences. They were expected to keep quiet about them and to forget them. People returning from more recent wars are expected to be open about their feelings. It is not to say one way is right and another wrong, but just to be aware of the cultural factors that affect how a narrative is developed and where it is used. For instance, a Second World War veteran may not be able to relate to his grandson or granddaughter serving in Iraq: the way they both think about support and 'opening up' may be very different because of the times in which each grew up and experienced active service.

Trying to create your own narrative

As we have said previously, this book is not intended to provide you with the answers to your reactions. It is meant to provide you with information so that you understand your situation more clearly. If you feel you may be seriously traumatized then you should seek professional help. The following is some guidance that may help those of you who are troubled by your memories of a traumatic incident, but feel able to deal with those memories. Please bear in mind that, if you start thinking deeply about what has happened to you, you may start to feel worse rather than better. This often happens, so you do need to be careful. If you have good social support, you should use it. If you do feel worse, you should go to the doctor and obtain treatment. The following guidelines are intended to help you make sense of your experiences, but not as an alternative to therapy if that is what you need. We do think, though, that someone who is prepared to buy this book and read it this far is likely to gain from attempting to tell his or her own story.

Guidelines

A story has a number of characteristics, for example a beginning, a middle and an end. It also has a narrative sense; it makes sense if someone reads it, it has a purpose. In order to write a sensible narrative about a traumatic experience you do not have to be a novelist or even a good writer: it is more about being able to write down the components of the story and put them together in a logical order. The difficulty is that your memories and feelings may be disjointed, unclear; you may not be able to remember key aspects of the event. Don't worry about that. It will come later – if it needs to. Another thing you should know from the outset is that the story will not be fixed. You may write for a week, as Tricia did, described at the beginning of the chapter, and you may think you have sorted things out very well; but traumatic memories have a way of returning in the future, sometimes unexpectedly. You need to keep this in mind. What you are trying to do is learn to manage your memories, learn to cope with them when they do appear.

To turn to the practical aspects of creating your story, the following guidelines are just that: guidelines. They are not meant to be rigorously applied. You may find better ways of telling your story. They are devised to provide prompts when you are stuck, or guidance about where you might want to go next. Each part should be completed in as much detail as possible.

1 Describe the traumatic incident in as much detail as you can. Where did it take place? What happened exactly? Think about the people involved: describe what they looked like, what they did, what they said. If it is the kind of trauma that involves multiple events, think of the one with the most painful or detailed memories. Describe more than one inci-

dent if there are several that are particularly painful. It is up to you. The more you can describe an event, the better it will be in the end. Put the event into context. What were you doing before? What had you planned to do?

2 Describe your thoughts and your feelings in relation to the event at the time it happened and immediately after. Can you link those thoughts and feelings to particular aspects of the event, or to the actions of an individual? Try to remember as many thoughts and feelings as possible. You may have felt fear or anger. Describe it and describe why you felt it. You may have been shocked by what someone did. Why was that? It may seem obvious, but write it down anyway.

3 Describe your thoughts and feelings as they have developed and changed – or as they have stayed the same – since the traumatic event. What do you think about the people involved? Do you still feel anger or fear? Try and explain why you think this might be.

4 Did your behaviour change after the traumatic event? In what ways? Think about how you have changed in relation to what you personally do differently, and also try and think about how you have changed – if you have changed – towards other people.

5 How have you managed to cope with your memories, feelings and thoughts about the traumatic event? Perhaps you feel you haven't coped. Describe this in detail. Why haven't you coped? What coping mechanisms have worked better than others? Do you feel you have social support? If so, from whom? How and why does it work? Have you relied on drink or drugs to help you keep going? Describe this in detail.

6 Over the time since the traumatic event, have you changed the way you think about it, or the way you think about other people or the world in general? Describe these.

7 How would you like to be able to deal with the traumatic event? How would you like your behaviour, thoughts and

feelings to be changed? What can you do to make this happen (apart from writing this account)? Think about the big changes you would like, but also the little things, because these are often the easier things to actually change.

8 When you have completed your account, put it to one side for the day, come back to it the following day, read it, and add or change any details you think need changing. Try to come back to the account regularly, every day at first and then perhaps less often, because it is likely that the act of writing the account has made you emotional. Over time you are likely to change fewer details.

9 Share the account if there is someone you trust. If not, keep it to yourself. It is your account.

You should find that over time the very act of writing in detail about these various elements of the traumatic event does help you put things into context and does help you develop your own narrative, your own understanding of what you have been through. Remember, though, that it is not an alternative to therapy and it is not suitable for everyone.

In the next chapters we will explore the various forms of therapy that are available to people who are traumatized. It is helpful to have some idea of what is on offer when you go for assistance.

7

How do we treat post-traumatic stress disorder?

There are many methods used to treat PTSD. This chapter will examine some of the key themes to give you some understanding of what happens in therapy, so that if you choose to use it your experiences will make sense. The methods vary in effectiveness depending on both the particular treatment and the individual. Some treatments are more effective for some people; others are more effective for others.

The treatment of mental health issues is complex. There is a wide range of disorders that affect the mind and behaviour in many different ways, from relatively straightforward cases of generalized anxiety or depression through to complex psychoses such as schizophrenia. The phenomenon of mental health has been studied using modern scientific methods since the late nineteenth century, when people such as Charcot, Breuer and Freud provided detailed case reports on people with mental health disorders.

Mental health can be stigmatizing in many societies. This is often because people do not understand why others behave as they do. Physical illness is relatively easy to understand. Someone has a fever, a blocked nose, a cancerous growth, and the treatments are often (but by no means always) straightforward: apply drug treatment and the person gets better. Also, the symptoms of physical illnesses are generally coherent, a set of symptoms usually group together to form a syndrome, and a doctor can assess the symptoms, provide a diagnosis, and suggest a form of treatment.

Mental health is often not like that. We do classify mental disorders in the same way as physical ones, but this approach does not always work. While physical illnesses relate to the environment – perhaps there is a virus in the population, or someone smokes which leads to cancer – mental health disorders often interact more closely with the person's physical and social environment. This can make them more difficult to treat.

As we have seen, PTSD is by definition linked with the environment, with the traumatic event itself, which is included as a diagnostic criterion. As we have also seen, the response to a traumatic event is complex, and the symptoms are not all part of the PTSD construct. Many people diagnosed with PTSD are also diagnosed with other disorders such as depression or substance abuse. For this reason, before someone receives treatment he or she is given a thorough assessment, to find out exactly what the situation is. In this chapter we discuss a number of methods of treatment so that you will be aware of the kinds of help you may receive, and so that you can be more knowledgeable when a therapist discusses the possibilities with you. It is quite common for someone with a complex trauma reaction to receive different kinds of treatment for different symptoms or at different points in the course of the treatment. This is important; if you are to be treated effectively, you may need different forms of treatment at different points. One type of treatment does not necessarily work for all your symptoms.

Before we go any further, it is worth taking note of the evidence regarding the effectiveness of the various forms of treatment and examining the limitations of that evidence. The NICE guidelines, published in 2005, recommend cognitive behavioural therapy (CBT) as being the most effective form of treatment, along with eye movement desensitization and reprocessing (EMDR). This is not to say that other forms of treatment don't work, just that the evidence we have does not clearly show that they are effective. Also bear in mind that no single treatment is suited to everyone. While CBT may be effective for some, the style of treatment may be too difficult for many people to manage. Some may prefer (and benefit from) a more relaxed analytic approach. This demonstrates the importance of receiving treatment from a fully qualified practitioner who can serve your needs best. It also highlights the importance of the initial assessment.

Treatment for traumatic stress is not about a reversion to the time before the traumatic event, and it is not a cure that sorts out all the problems: treatment is used to help traumatized people cope with their traumatic memories, to help them develop an understanding of their own strengths and weaknesses regarding the ways they think about their experiences, to break the close bond between memory and emotion, and to develop coping strategies to deal with any future issues, e.g. memories, which may emerge. Treatment is designed to help people move on from being haunted by the past to becoming engaged with the present and the future, and to place the traumatic event or period as an historical event. At its most basic, treatment is about the deconditioning of anxiety and altering the way people see themselves, increasing personal integrity and control, and establishing meaningful relationships with others.

Variety of therapists

Pete, the Falklands veteran we met in Chapter 3, eventually realized, with a bit of persuasion from his parents, that he needed help – this was the first stage in dealing with his situation. He went to his GP, who sent him to a counsellor. One meeting was enough. Pete didn't turn up to the second one. There seemed to be no point. The GP then sent him to a clinical psychologist. Again, this did not work. Pete just did not get on with him. The GP then realized what the problem was; it wasn't the type of treatment, but the type of therapist. The GP contacted Combat Stress, a charity that looks after veterans with mental health disorders. Pete was visited by one of their welfare officers (himself ex-services) and received treatment from a clinical psychologist who was also a veteran.

> This worked. Pete trusted the therapist, feeling that the therapist understood him because he had been through similar experiences himself (whether he had or not didn't matter). Pete responded to treatment and made a steady recovery.

This shows that it is not only the type of training a therapist has that matters (we discuss this below) but also specifically who that therapist is and his or her personal background. The therapist–client relationship is a subtle one, full of emotion, dependent on trust, so each person must get the right therapist.

There is a wide range of therapists who may treat people affected by traumatic stress. In the UK, the most common are clinical psychologists, who are trained in a variety of techniques. They may use CBT, EMDR, psychoanalytic psychotherapy, humanistic therapy or any of a number of other techniques. Many specialize in particular forms of treatment. Clinical psychologists work both within the National Health Service and privately. They are generally the best-trained therapists, having undergone a three-year taught doctorate after their first degree. Unfortunately, the waiting list to see a clinical psychologist can be very long when referred by your GP. Clinical psychologists are not currently able to prescribe drugs, and if your symptoms are severe enough to require drug treatment you may be referred to a psychiatrist, a medical doctor who specializes in mental health and who can also provide psychological therapies. There are many other types of therapist, some of whom work within the NHS and some of whom work privately: mental health nurses working within the NHS; cognitive behavioural therapists (who have their own respected professional body, the British Association of Behavioural and Cognitive Psychotherapies or BABCP); psychoanalytic therapists; humanist therapists; and many others.

If you are not being referred within the NHS you should ensure that a therapist you contact is bone fide by checking whether he or she belongs to a respected professional body and is fully licensed to provide therapy. Unfortunately, while most

are very well trained and have a great deal of expertise, the .
of psychotherapy is not yet fully professionalized; and soı.._
people do set themselves up as therapists without full training.

Initial assessment

Before any treatment can take place it is essential that a thorough
assessment is carried out to find out exactly what the situation
is. As we have seen, traumatic stress is a complex disorder that
presents in many different ways. There is usually no simple treatment solution. The therapist must find out the details of your
symptoms, and the context in which they are set. It is important
to look at the traumatic memories, the thoughts, beliefs, emotions
and feelings associated with these memories, and the behaviours
that are the consequences of these thoughts and feelings. The
therapist must also examine how you cope, how you appraise
situations, the support and help you are already receiving, and
whether this is effective. Trauma affects not only you but also
your family and friends, and so it is important the therapist
understands this social context. It is also the case that family and
friends can be the ones who will help you through your troubles.

In summary, some of the key areas that a therapist will ask
questions about include:

- the nature of the traumatic stressor
- your role in the event
- your thoughts and feelings about actions taken and not taken
- the effect of the trauma on your life and on those around you
- your personal perceptions of yourself and other people
- your exposure to previous traumatic events and prior psychiatric history
- your habitual coping styles and how these have changed as a
  result of the traumatic experience
- your level of cognitive functioning (e.g. your ability to think
  clearly, concentrate and solve the problems of everyday life)

- your personal strengths and weaknesses
- your medical, family and occupational history
- your cultural and religious beliefs
- your drug and alcohol use or misuse.

Treatment plan

Once the assessment is complete, a therapist will devise a treatment plan and discuss it with you. It is important that you are fully involved with the decisions regarding the type of treatment, as treatment can be difficult to deal with and you must be fully committed. There may be times when you are going to feel worse than you already do, and times when you despair that treatment is ever going to work, so you must be motivated to take part in the treatment and follow it through to completion.

The actual treatment will depend on the individual. For instance, there is little point in providing high levels of exposure to a memory for someone who is avoidant. There are practical issues to consider. If someone does not have a home and good access to food then that has to be dealt with first (this often applies to refugees). The plan will depend on whether the therapist thinks the client may be non-compliant, i.e. refusing to undertake certain treatment tasks. Also, there may be different types of treatment at different stages. For instance, someone who is extremely anxious may need drug treatment to deal with the anxiety before a talking therapy to deal with the causes of the anxiety. Someone who is avoidant may need to deal with relationship or emotional problems. In all, the treatment plan should be highly individual.

What kinds of treatment are available?

While we cannot look in detail at all the treatments available, we will consider some of the key ones. As already stated, this information is not intended to provide you with treatment, but to inform you of the treatments available, so you are better able to make choices in discussion with a therapist.

Cognitive and behavioural techniques

As mentioned earlier, cognitive behavioural therapy (CBT) is one of the most widely used and recommended types of treatment. It is not a single form of treatment but a wide range of techniques that are applied as appropriate to the situation. It is the most commonly used form of treatment in the UK, and its efficacy has been established through numerous studies. However, before you start thinking it is some kind of panacea that will help everyone, it is worth stating that while it is very beneficial for a lot of people, it does not work for everyone. It requires a lot of hard work on the part of the individual concerned, a lot of motivation and a level of self-awareness. The person must have the emotional strength to deal with the treatment.

There are a number of components to CBT, which are in the first place split into behavioural and cognitive techniques.

Behavioural techniques

These involve learning a range of skills to help you cope with the traumatic memory. They are mainly concerned with exposure (to reminders of the traumatic event) and anxiety management (to help you deal with these reminders effectively), and may include:

- breathing training to help you relax;
- reliving of the traumatic memory, basically going over the memory many times in order to gradually and carefully expose the self to the memory, which helps you get used to dealing with it. In conjunction with relaxation, this in itself can help you get used to your memories;
- exposure, whether in reality or imagined (e.g. through the use of pictures), to objects and situations that remind you

of the traumatic event. Again, in conjunction with relaxation, exposure can enable you to learn to deal with these reminders.

Behavioural techniques are very practical, and the evidence for their effectiveness is very good. They provide the skills to help you deal with everyday situations, to start to get on with your life again.

Cognitive techniques

Cognitive therapy is often used alongside behavioural techniques, because traumatized people do have thought-related problems as well as emotional and anxiety-related problems. Cognitive therapy teaches you to identify trauma-related unhelpful or distorted beliefs, and to challenge and modify them. It helps you to replace such distorted beliefs with more functional and helpful ones.

Albert Ellis, a psychologist from the USA who introduced rational emotive behaviour therapy, discussed what he called irrational beliefs that were associated with mental problems such as trauma. He provided a list of such beliefs that are commonly held by people. Some examples include:

- I must be competent and achieving, otherwise I am a worthless person.
- I cannot face life's responsibilities and difficulties, so it is easier to avoid them.
- I must be dependent on other people and I need them; I cannot run my own life.
- There is a right and precise solution to all problems, and it is awful if this solution cannot be found.

You will see that these are the kinds of beliefs we hold – if not these exact ones, then something similar. People who are traumatized often hold similar irrational beliefs about themselves, other people and the world, and cognitive techniques attempt to replace these beliefs with others that are more effective for dealing with the world.

Coping with negative thoughts

Cognitive techniques also help people cope with negative thoughts, e.g. 'I am worthless', 'I don't think I can cope with my job.' The therapist will work with you via a series of questions to address the kinds of thoughts that you are having. The questions may include:

- What is the evidence for the thought?
- What alternative views are there? How would someone else view it?
- What is the effect of thinking the way I do? Does it hinder me?
- Is my thinking realistic? Am I condemning myself on one event? Am I expecting myself to be perfect?
- What action can I take? How can I change my situation?

A CBT session

A typical CBT session may involve a number of activities. It may start with an assessment of the level of symptoms, to see whether they are decreasing. If not, a different strategy may be needed. It may then examine your homework (yes, you do homework with CBT!), which may have been keeping a diary, dealing with your family or practising anxiety reduction techniques. You will go through these and examine what worked and what didn't. You may work on relaxation skills, or on skills training relating to a particular dysfunctional belief (e.g. 'I am a useless person'). Finally, the session may involve setting new homework.

Varieties of CBT

There are many different forms of CBT. What we have just described is generalized CBT, which is effective not only for traumatic stress but also for conditions such as anxiety and depression, and even giving up smoking. There are also situation-specific forms of CBT, such as that proposed in 1992 by Patricia Resick and Monika Schnicke, two psychologists from the USA who designed a form of the treatment specifically for rape victims. The cognitive restructuring element, which identifies and modifies distorted beliefs, focuses on safety, trust, power, esteem and intimacy. For the exposure element, the person is expected to write a detailed account of the rape and to reread it several times during sessions. There is good evidence for the effectiveness of these kinds of trauma-specific CBT.

> Pete's therapist used CBT techniques with him to deal with his issues relating to anger and to guilt. The therapist taught Pete to relax, and showed him how to employ this skill when he felt himself getting tense in a situation. This – so both hoped – would reduce the chances of Pete getting into a fight. The therapist also worked on Pete's beliefs about why he had such anger with everyone, helping him to realize that this was something he could work out and that, if he stopped being angry with himself for missing the homecoming after the Falklands, his overall anger would diminish. Pete was irrationally angry with the world for something that wasn't the world's fault! Pete also had difficulties relating to esteem and intimacy, and CBT helped him along the road to understanding these reactions and dealing with them.

EMDR

Eye movement desensitization and reprocessing (EMDR) was introduced in the 1990s by Francine Shapiro. It was initially treated with some scepticism, but has now been accepted as a very effective and rapid treatment, though there is still a need to see whether it is effective over the long term. It has many similarities to CBT, but involves a key difference: The therapist moves a finger (or a pencil) from side to side in front of the client's face. Clients must keep their head still and follow the finger with their eyes, while at the same time thinking about the traumatic memory. The image of the traumatic event is frozen, and that is why people continually relive it. People generate vivid images, thoughts, feelings and body sensations associated with the trauma. They are asked within the treatment session to evaluate the aversive qualities of these and replace them with alternative cognitions, at the same time as tracking the therapist's finger. This leads to a rapid reduction in the negative symptoms. The mechanism for this is as yet unknown, but it is effective with many people. It is quite possible that the rapid eye movements may deflect attention from the anxiety relating to thinking about the trauma, leading to the person having a more detached perspective on the event, which in itself leads to resolution.

The treatment sessions for EMDR follow a similar pattern to those for CBT, where the client history is initially obtained, a treatment plan is developed, followed by a series of sessions involving the reprocessing and desensitization, a consideration of bodily sensations such as tension and anxiety, and closure.

Closure

Most forms of treatment do not end with closure, as the person may have further issues arising at some point in the future. It is important for many types of treatment that there is a fixed number of treatment sessions so the person does not become dependent on the therapist, and is prepared for the treatment sessions to finish. This is different from some psychoanalytic techniques (discussed below), where treatment may continue for years.

Narrative techniques

As we discussed in Chapter 6, narrative techniques are being increasingly used to treat traumatized people. In one way, all types of talking therapy aim to help the person develop a narrative or a story about the traumatic experiences, to make sense of them. At its simplest, narrative refers to stories and story development, and people are encouraged to develop their own stories about their traumatic experiences to help them put these stories into meaningful contexts. There are a number of specific techniques available, and there is some evidence for their effectiveness. We introduced narrative exposure therapy (NET) in the previous chapter, as a good example of narrative techniques. While it is just one technique among several narrative approaches, there is good evidence that it works. NET was designed to deal with the problems people face resulting from organized violence. It has mainly been used with refugee groups, but it can be used with other people who have experienced traumatic events. It is based on CBT (discussed above) and testimony therapy, which is a form of treatment involved with getting the person to provide a witness statement regarding his or her experiences that can be used in a court of law. The aim of NET is to produce a document that describes a person's experiences and that can eventually be used in a court as evidence against the perpetrators of a crime. It also aims to help people cope with their traumatic memories.

The person is asked, in a safe environment away from the scene of the traumatic experience, to talk about his or her worst memory of the event. Through a process of developing the narrative over several sessions, the person tries to weave the 'hot implicit memories' (i.e. the traumatic memories) into 'cool declarative memories' (i.e. memories that can more easily be dealt with). This leads to habituation, the ability to come to term with the memory.

Proponents of NET claim that it has a number of therapeutic elements. These include:

- the active reconstruction of the autobiographical memory
- prolonged exposure to 'hot spots' and the full activation of the fear memory through narration
- linking the original context of where the memory was acquired and the re-emergence of conditioned emotional responses

- the cognitive re-evaluation of behaviour and beliefs (reprocessing of memories)
- regaining personal dignity through testifying.

NET involves a series of sessions, during which people develop their narration. In the first session, the individual is diagnosed through a series of measures and receives psychoeducation, which involves describing his or her reactions, learning that these reactions are normal and legitimate, and having the therapeutic procedure explained. In the second session, the person provides a life narrative from birth through to and including the traumatic experience. This provides a context for the third and subsequent sessions, which involve rereading the narrative and developing it as necessary. The final session involves rereading the narrative and signing the completed document, which can then, if appropriate, be used in a court of law as evidence against a perpetrator of the crime.

There are many other narrative techniques available, but they all use similar principles, helping the person develop a story of the traumatic event.

Drug treatments

A wide range of psychopharmacological approaches are used to treat traumatic stress including, among others, anxiolytics and antidepressants. It is important to know something of what these drugs do – not only which symptoms they treat, but also their potential side effects and long-term effects. Drugs are usually used to treat traumatic stress when the person has extremely serious symptoms, such as very high levels of anxiety. In these cases it often helps to prescribe drugs in order that these symptoms can be controlled and the person is then able to undertake a talking therapy: that is, drug treatments are often used to make psychotherapy more effective.

We cannot establish a single pattern of drug treatment as the symptoms of traumatic stress are complicated and individual.

There are multiple symptoms, and a particular drug may only be effective for one of them. While several drugs may be effective, there are only a few controlled studies to demonstrate their effectiveness with traumatic stress.

Some of the drugs that are used to treat traumatic stress include the following:

- Antidepressants, such as monoamine oxidase inhibitors, improve sleep, diminish the physiological startle response and decrease intrusive thoughts.
- Adrenergic blocking agents, such as propranolol or clonidine, decrease physiological arousal and the startle response, and reduce the number of nightmares and intrusive thoughts.
- Antipsychotics, also known as neuroleptics, are used rarely and then only in very severe cases. Low doses of neuroleptics have been shown to control severe flashbacks and agitation.
- Lithium carbonate reduces anger and anxiety and can help people sleep better.
- The minor tranquillizers such as diazepam and the benzo-diazapines can control anger, but there is a high risk of dependence.
- Prozac and other similar drugs (selective seratonin reuptake inhibitors, or SSRIs) are useful just after the event for controlling the formation of traumatic memories.
- D-cycloserine (DCS) is generally used to treat tuberculosis, but like many drugs has been found to have properties which reduce other symptoms. It inhibits fear receptors and helps people to deal more constructively with their traumatic memories, to 'unlearn' the fear response. An experiment was carried out where people were injected with DCS half an hour before receiving exposure therapy, and this was shown to help improve the effectiveness of the exposure therapy.
- Yohimbine has been tested over the last few years with people who are traumatized. It helps facilitate the recall of traumatic

memories, and because of this has been shown to be useful in conjunction with psychotherapy. Unfortunately it can have severe side effects, such as causing anxiety.

The use of drugs is complex and depends on the needs of the individual, as determined by the assessment of a qualified practitioner. It may be that in certain circumstances taking a drug which produces side effects is more beneficial than not receiving drug treatment at all.

Psychological debriefing

This is a widely used, and often controversial, set of techniques. There are various types of psychological debriefing (e.g. critical incident stress debriefing, multiple stress debriefing), but they share many characteristics. They all have a structured format, and are formal meetings after a traumatic event. Psychological debriefing has its origins in the First World War treatment known as PIE (proximity, immediacy, expectancy), which we met in Chapter 1: traumatized soldiers were treated near to the front line (proximity), as soon as they experienced symptoms (immediacy) and with the knowledge that after treatment they would resume their normal duties with their unit (expectancy). In the Second World War a debriefing technique was introduced where it was suggested that if a soldier experienced a single day's fighting, then that individual would need seven hours' debriefing. The procedure was meant to be spiritually purging, and was a simple intervention that could be undertaken by the troops' commander.

Modern psychological debriefing is an intervention conducted shortly after a traumatic event, where those involved are invited to either an individual session or, more commonly, a group session, during which they are encouraged to talk about their experiences and to receive information about the 'normal reactions' to traumatic events. The purpose of debriefing is to reduce the long-term problems which may emerge weeks or months after the event. It has been used with different groups, from emergency workers to disaster victims. It is intended to help people normalize their initial reactions and to start to think about the feelings and emotions associated with the event.

The key elements of debriefing are:

- an outline of the aim of the session
- respect for each person's experience and feelings
- suspension of judgement for the duration of the debriefing
- slow sequential exposition of the event, leading to cognitive reconstruction
- recognition of grief
- enabling an emotional response.

As an example of a technique, Jeffrey Mitchell of the University of Maryland described critical incident stress debriefing, which has seven phases:

1 a statement of the confidentiality of the meeting, and an outline of the session, that this is just a discussion, not psychotherapy; people are encouraged to talk, but are not forced to do so;
2 a statement of the facts of the event;
3 thoughts about the meaning of the event;
4 reactions and emotions (this tends to be the longest part of the meeting);
5 recognizing and acknowledging symptoms of distress;
6 teaching normality;
7 summary.

It is difficult to assess whether psychological debriefing really works. It is essentially a good idea, enabling people to start to build their story or narrative about the event and to understand their feelings and responses. A group session also provides social

support. One scientific review attempted to assess the effectiveness of these techniques, and summarized the findings from six
studies. Two showed that debriefing was effective, two showed it
did more harm than good, and two showed mixed results! This
is probably because, like any psychological therapy, debriefing
will work for some people and not for others. Some people like
to talk about their stressful experiences, others do not; and this
difference should always be respected.

Family therapy

Family therapy is a form of treatment that recognizes the importance of the person's interactions within the family, and how
these interactions can both help recovery and hinder it. It is
well known that the best form of help a person can get is social
support, and usually the most effective social support is provided
by the family. If the family members (wife, husband or partner,
children or parents) do not know how to react, and behave in
ways that do not alleviate the symptoms or perhaps make them
worse, it can be helpful to see the therapist together. With the
help of the therapist, the family can understand the dynamics
of the way they interact, and can learn to interact with each
other more effectively. For instance, a spouse might criticize a
traumatized person for not 'behaving normally', provoking an
impatient response and, in the end, an argument. If the spouse
can be helped to understand this, and if the traumatized person
can understand why the spouse is behaving like this, then they
can both learn to be more understanding of each other. They
may learn helping strategies: for instance, when they recognize
an argument is developing, they should stop and make a cup of
tea, or go out for a walk, or whatever is most effective for them.
There is good evidence that family therapy can work in trauma
cases, but each member has to accept that it can make a positive
difference.

Other techniques

There are many other psychological therapies used to treat traumatic stress. The evidence for these techniques is at best mixed. You have to bear in mind that while one technique may work for many people, no technique works for everyone.

Two of the most common are the various forms of humanist-existential therapy and psychoanalysis. Psychoanalysis has been used since the days of Freud, and exists in numerous forms. It tends to take much longer than other types of treatment. Many people undergo years of such treatment, and there is no evidence regarding whether or not it works. Like many things, if you think it is doing you good then it probably is, but research does not show any improvement better than chance. Existential-humanist approaches have been popular since the 1960s and essentially try to help people make sense of their experiences – again, this is a form of narrative development.

Conclusion

Clinical psychologists are likely to employ techniques from across the range of therapies. If there is a psychoanalytic technique that they think might work then they will use it, perhaps in the context of other cognitive and behavioural techniques. Given the complexity of the response to traumatic events, it is beneficial to have a therapist who is trained across the spectrum of techniques and can apply what should work best for each individual. As we stated earlier, while the evidence for the therapies is at best mixed, CBT techniques tend to show the best effects – at least with some people. The evidence is weak concerning the very long-term (e.g. years) benefits of treatment.

Treatment for traumatic stress is not about a return to the pre-trauma state: it is about helping you to cope with your memories by learning a series of skills. It is also there to help you deal with the emotions and thoughts that you have regarding the traumatic event.

8

Problems faced by family and friends

After Geoff and Sandy's car accident, there were consequences not only for the two of them but also for others. While we have seen that Sandy confided in her friend, Geoff did not, and nor did he appear to have other ways of coping, so PTSD symptoms developed. They had a little boy, Ryan, who worshipped his father, but once Geoff started to have problems this relationship suffered. Geoff stopped responding to Ryan and did not seem to care as much, and both Sandy and Ryan noticed it. Sandy tried to intervene but it did not help, and Ryan became very upset and started to avoid his father. It wasn't until the three of them went to family therapy, and the family therapist helped Geoff see that his emotional difficulties were disturbing his relationship with Ryan, that things started to improve. Indeed, in the end it was Ryan who helped Geoff recover from his PTSD, making him see the negative consequences of the disorder and encouraging him to go for professional help.

PTSD is a terrible disorder that has severe consequences not only for the individual but also for those around. Chapter 5 considered the importance of social support for the person with PTSD; this chapter will explore the difficulties experienced by those providing the social support. They are often faced with not being able to understand why a person is behaving in a particular way, why love has been withdrawn or why someone is angry. Someone with PTSD does not always display symptoms that are clearly linked to the traumatic experience. For instance, an ex-soldier traumatized by war may not display any symptoms until several years after leaving the forces. When symptoms do emerge, they may appear as marriage problems or issues relating to work. It is important that the carer can establish the true cause of the situation, as it is only then that the problems can be addressed effectively.

Friends and family of a traumatized person are themselves liable to experience symptoms that are described as secondary traumatic stress, the result of being distressed by someone else's responses to traumatic experiences. This chapter will outline the evidence relating to this subject in order to make readers aware of the potential problems.

The family situation

Traumatized people can be difficult to live with. As we have seen, the symptoms of psychological trauma are not like most other health problems: they are complex, difficult to deal with and extremely distressing. People who are traumatized experience a wide range of intense emotions, from fear and sadness through to anger and rage. They can be impossible to live with, and trauma can break up a family unless the person seeks help. We would recommend that if you are having family problems then you should immediately seek professional advice. This can be difficult to do, but it will be worth it in the end. We briefly discussed family therapy in the previous chapter, and this may be suitable if you are experiencing difficulties. See Useful addresses for details of relevant organizations, but also go and see your GP, who may be aware of local organizations.

The first thing to do is try and understand what the traumatized person is experiencing. Hopefully this book will have helped you towards that. Understanding why a person is behaving in a particular way is the first step towards being able to help, rather than becoming involved in arguments, which can escalate into real long-term relationship problems. Unfortunately there are many examples where a traumatized person has become violent and has ended up in the law courts. There are many traumatized people who are in prison because they became violent as a result of their symptoms. In some cases, the violence arises because the people around 'do not understand' what someone has been through, and the individual becomes frustrated and may lash out. There is no simple solution to this. Someone who has been through a traumatic situation has almost by definition had an experience that the people around them will not and cannot fully understand. That is not to say that people do not have sympathy and want to help. This chapter has to address both the traumatized person and the people around him or her; the traumatized person needs to try and understand that those around are attempting to help, but equally that it is difficult for them to see a loved one behaving so strangely, so emotionally, perhaps so aggressively. Family and friends need to understand that it is sometimes very difficult for traumatized people to control the way they behave at times, that if they lash out this is often beyond their control, and that the regrets they later express are genuine.

We require safety, and in extreme cases where someone is being aggressive then that means the family members – including children – may need protection. They may need to move out, hopefully on a temporary basis, until the traumatized person is able to manage and control his or her emotions and behaviour. Contact your local social services or your GP. There may also be local charities that can help.

Fortunately, most people who are traumatized are not violent, but they do find it hard to contain their emotions. One of the difficulties for family and friends is when a person appears to withdraw love and cease to care for them. As we have seen, emotional numbing is a common symptom of trauma. This is where difficulty dealing with the intense fear, horror or helplessness associated with memories causes the individual to apparently shut down his or her emotions altogether; not only does this block intense negative emotions, but it also means that the person is unable to experience the most positive emotions of love, joy and happiness. This can be very difficult for the people around. The traumatized person does not do this deliberately; it is an automatic defence against the awfulness of the traumatic memories.

Members of the same household as the traumatized person may need to learn skills for dealing with the person's symptoms. This is why family therapy can be effective, as it focuses on the specific areas of difficulty within the relationships. The skills may be as simple as keeping out of the way of the traumatized person when she is angry, making a cup of tea when he is upset, or suggesting they go out for a walk. It is not possible to provide a comprehensive list here, as there are so many different ways of helping and everyone is different. It may be best to work out the best options between yourselves, if that is possible. Sometimes this may work better if there is a mediator. It is always best to discuss ways of dealing with the symptoms when the person is not experiencing them rather than try to have a discussion in the heat of the moment.

Protection against traumatic memories

If people describe their traumatic memories in detail to their loved ones, this can be distressing to the loved ones. It is true, though, that many people who are traumatized do not want to share their memories in this way, perhaps aware of the potential psychological damage it may cause. As discussed in Chapter 5, research with Second World War veterans found that many of them had never discussed their experiences in detail with their families, perhaps because they wanted to protect them and to ensure the home was a safe place, away from traumatic memories. These veterans tended to share their memories with others who had been through similar experiences. This is common in traumatic stress.

Secondary traumatic stress

This is a growing area of research which examines the symptoms that people associated with the traumatized people might experience. A number of terms are used, including 'secondary traumatic stress' or 'vicarious trauma', but these are slightly misleading in that people do not generally become traumatized through the experiences of others. It is not that those with PTSD necessarily share their traumatic memories, but that their behaviour can be changed so much that it affects their relationships with others, which itself has an impact on those other people.

Much of the research has been conducted using therapists who treat traumatized people. It is often found that, over time, such therapists may experience a form of burnout, where they become deeply tired, distressed and unable to continue with their work. Most therapists have supervision sessions with colleagues to discuss the stories they have heard and their experiences in the therapy room, which does help reduce any developing problems. Effectively, such supervision is formalized social support – which we know is the best thing to protect against the effects of stress and trauma.

Other research has been conducted on the families of those who have been traumatized, particularly the impact on children and grandchildren. It is clear that being traumatized can affect the way you bring up children, not necessarily by traumatizing them but by behaving in different – often subtly different – ways. For instance, you may not allow your children the freedom they need in order to develop fully, being over-protective because you, the parent, are frightened of society.

Inevitably, a person who is traumatized is going to affect those around. Someone who is traumatized can display a range of symptoms, from anger and rage through to depression and social withdrawal. In extreme cases, people may attack their own families, or they may stop talking to them. Barriers are often drawn up, as though those who are traumatized are trying to protect themselves and others from their traumatic memories. Unfortunately, this protection, while well meant, can have terrible effects on the people around them.

One role of family therapy can be to help with the secondary problems of traumatic stress. If a child, spouse or partner is affected by the behaviour of the traumatized person, family therapists can provide appropriate assistance; by helping both the traumatized person and the family to understand what is happening and to develop the skills to stop it happening in future, the therapist can help people start to live a more normal life again. It is often hard living with a traumatized person; in some ways the trauma is always shared, though the normal channels of communication (talking, doing things together) may be temporarily closed. Therapy, and simply being aware of the reactions that are caused by the trauma, can help deal with the problems.

9

Growing through experience

Tricia, after dealing with the worst of her symptoms relating to her rape, decided that she wanted to do more. She realized that the experience had changed her and that she had learned a lot during the process of recovery, and she wanted to help others in similar circumstances. After she had recovered and was back at work, she decided to contact Victim Support, which provides help for victims of crime. After ensuring she was well, Victim Support provided training and Tricia worked for them, specializing in rape victims. With her first-hand knowledge, Tricia was able to provide appropriate support to others.

This chapter will explore trauma from an alternative perspective, that of resilience and growth. Research has shown that many people who experience traumatic events come out of it feeling that in some way they have benefited from the experience, that they have grown wiser or that they are psychologically stronger. This chapter explores how and why that might happen, and how people can help themselves to experience growth.

This is a change from earlier chapters, which have generally focused on the negative side of traumatic stress, something that is of course dominant in most people most of the time. This chapter is here to show that, in the end, at least for some people, there is a more positive side to traumatic stress, one where people believe that they have learned something profound from their experiences. After all, traumatic stress is a profound experience that is concerned with the actual threat to one's life, so it is not surprising that such experiences make people think differently about their lives.

Another factor that is important here is what happens after a traumatic event. There is often an assumption that most people are traumatized. This is wrong: most people are not traumatized by such experiences. People may well be upset, they may have difficult emotional memories, but if these are controllable then they are not traumatized. It is normal to be upset when a life-threatening event occurs.

What is growth?

It may be helpful to look back at some earlier ideas to illustrate what we mean by growth. This is not a modern concept. Positive changes after a traumatic experience have long been recognized outside psychology. Many of our religions are founded on learning from human suffering: Buddhism originated as an attempt to come to terms with suffering; Christianity teaches redemption through the suffering of Jesus. Within literature, the concept of tragedy itself is a means – through novels or plays – to show that we can learn from tragic events. A tragedy in terms of literature is a narrative with several stages: the precipitant, which might be some act of horror or shame (the traumatic or tragedic event), followed by suffering (traumatic stress), leading to some insight or learning, some increase in knowledge or understanding, and finishing with an affirmation that life is worthwhile, that death has some meaning, that the human spirit has dignity. We can see, through the study of terrible events, from war and rape through chronic illness, cancer and HIV, that people do go through similar stages – not everyone, and the stages are not necessarily clear, but a narrative of a traumatic event will in some way have these elements.

In recent years, psychologists have introduced the idea of positive psychology. It is really a reaction against psychology focusing on the negative, on pathology. We have clinical psychologists who deal with mental health problems, occupational psychologists who deal with companies that do not work effectively, health psychologists who look at physical health problems, so perhaps we need positive psychologists, who look at the happier things in life, to show how, for most people most of the time, life is positive – and it can be again for people who have been traumatized. Positive psychology focuses on concepts such as hope, wisdom, creativity, courage, responsibility and perseverance, the positive aspects that make humans so resilient and show that life is worth living. These concepts are often ignored in psychology.

Terminology

The concept of growth after trauma has been around since the 1990s, and there are a number of terms that are used to describe it, including 'post-traumatic growth', 'stress-related growth', 'perceived benefits', 'thrivings', 'blessings', 'positive by-products' and 'positive readjustment'. According to the psychologists Alex Linley and Stephen Joseph, such growth is concerned with changes that propel the individual to a higher level of functioning.

Prevalence

It is all very well saying that people can grow from their experiences, but how many people actually do? This is a difficult question to answer because it is impossible to define completely what we mean by growth. Researchers and therapists disagree. As we have seen, they use different terminology which means different things. When they measure growth (which seems an odd concept – it is not clear that you can use a questionnaire to provide a final number indicating the extent of growth) they measure it in different ways. Nevertheless, Linley and Joseph reviewed 39 studies and found huge discrepancies, from one study that found only 3 per cent experiencing growth after bereavement to another studying showing 98 per cent experiencing it after breast cancer. Of course, it is extremely likely not only that there are methodological problems, such as defining the concept and measuring growth, but also that people are more or less likely to experience growth after different kinds of events. People who survive breast cancer may well be encouraged to experience growth because they have survived, while if someone has lost a husband or wife then life may seem more hopeless and the widow(er) may find it very difficult to experience hope and 'growth'.

Existential change

We briefly discussed existentialism in Chapter 7. Existential growth relates to the work on narratives (see Chapter 6), and is concerned with how trauma is resolved through existentialist change, i.e. making fundamental changes to the meaning of one's life. This might involve a fundamental change of identity, actually feeling that you have become a different person and are no longer the one who was traumatized but someone who has moved beyond the trauma. Existential change is also about strengthening your personal control and autonomy, becoming an independent person who controls your own life, rather than being controlled by others. It is about having a greater understanding of the world, and how you as an individual can relate to that world.

Treatment

As we have seen in earlier chapters, positive change can be developed within the concept of treatment. While there is more of an emphasis on positive change in therapies such as existential, humanist or narrative, all treatments are concerned with such change. It is critical to develop a more positive view of the self, for example through CBT, where the cognitive elements may be concerned with changing one's beliefs.

What characteristics predict growth?

There are a number of personal and social characteristics that seem to predict whether growth will occur. Perhaps the most important is the way the person appraises his or her situation. It may seem surprising, but those who perceive greater threat and harm at the time of the traumatic event may experience greater growth. This may be because these people have a more realistic view of the danger of the situation, and may be more realistic in the way that they develop afterwards. This may link to people with greater cognitive abilities reporting more growth. The evidence does suggest that younger adults and those with a higher level of education and income are more likely to experience growth. Some work has been done with personality and growth, and it was found that people who are neurotic are less likely to experience growth, while extroverts and those who are conscientious are more likely to experience growth. The trouble is that these variables are probably mixed up, and the results are never very clear.

In terms of coping, as we discussed in Chapter 5, many kinds of effective mechanisms are associated with growth. These include both problem-focused and emotion-focused coping, along with religion as a source of strength and meaning. People who are able to process the trauma-related information, who try to develop the narrative, also seem to be more likely to experience growth. The important point here is that it is effective coping that is important; it doesn't seem to matter how you cope, as long as you are coping effectively – which is a bit of a circular argument.

How is growth related to other characteristics?

People have tried to work out how growth is related to other aspects of traumatic stress, and what appears to be important is both the effectiveness of trying to think through your memories and make sense of them ('cognitive processing'), and also having effective social support. Social support, as we have seen, does not necessarily mean having a lot of friends: it is about how you *perceive* your interactions with your friends. If you are able to discuss things with them, or accept their advice, or just get on with your lives together, then you are more likely to be able to deal with your traumatic memories and your emotions. The idea of resilience is also important, a sort of inner strength that enables you to put up with the stress and trauma of life and get on with things. Resilience is probably negatively related to the expectation in society that people should experience problems after a traumatic event. Clearly, the more resilient you are, the better able you will be to cope.

Back to narrative

We want to argue here that the key to this is the narrative, discussed in Chapter 6. We know that among people who deal effectively with traumatic stress there is a massive rewriting of the life story after the traumatic event. It is not just that they try to get back their old life and their old ways of thinking: there is a more dramatic and serious change. The meaning of life itself can be reconstructed, and during this reconstruction, if it is effective, then people will fundamentally change the way they think, will resolve emotional issues arising from the traumatic experience, and hence will experience growth.

The psychologist Robert Neimeyer provided an example of what he called a 'disruptive narrative' regarding how a person can work through a trauma to experience growth.

> Sally experienced the death of her brother in the World Trade Center in 2001 in New York, USA. She was talking to him on the telephone after the plane had hit, and tried to talk him down the stairs as he tried to escape. She then heard a loud rumbling sound and the phone went dead. The tower had collapsed, so she had been talking to her brother at the point of his death.
>
> Sally's immediate reaction was the classic trauma response, with the disruption of thought and the fragmentation of memories. She was flooded with imagery for months; she had intrusive memories not only of her own but of others' grief; she constantly recollected the last hour

of her brother's life. Over time she began to obsessively piece together the fragments from the media to try to make out the story as it really happened. This was – understandably – a complex grief reaction, followed by a developing narrative that enabled Sally to have a more complex world view. She acknowledged the reality of death in a way she hadn't before, at the same time acknowledging the reality of death and human vulnerability. While the whole process took many months, Sally came to admit that she had learned a great deal about life because of the experience.

Another way in which narratives can get in the way of developing growth is what Neimeyer calls 'dissociated narratives'. An example of this is provided by Jane, whose husband committed suicide, but who could not acknowledge the fact, because she thought it would be her fault if he had committed suicide. She kept the fact of the suicide separate to the story that she told people about his death – she said it was an accident – so she was unable to acknowledge the reality of the suicide to the public world, to her friends and acquaintances, and it wasn't until she was able to do this that she was able to come to terms with the death, to develop the narrative and learn to live with the suicide.

A final kind of problem narrative that gets in the way of growth is what Neimeyer calls the 'dominant narrative'. This is where society has 'preferred accounts' of an event, as in the example of Julie.

Julie had had breast cancer that was successfully treated. Unfortunately, Julie experienced a number of psychological symptoms relating to the breast cancer. When her therapist explored this, he found that Julie thought of herself only as a cancer patient, not as a fully rounded human being. Through the course of the cancer, she had 'learned' to become a cancer patient, accepting treatment, accepting the risks of success and failure, reading all about the cancer, etc. She had immersed herself so much in this that she was finding it difficult to recover. Once this was acknowledged, she started to have more positive experiences and began to live her life more fully again, regaining her former happiness and also experiencing growth in the knowledge that she was strong enough to deal with one of the worst things the world can throw at you.

Julie's story illustrates how the dominant societal narrative (cancer patient) can stop someone from developing his or her own personal narrative, and inhibits psychological growth.

In an ideal world – which is very rare in the case of trauma – post-traumatic growth involves seeking a new sense of coherence from the disorganizing life experience of the trauma. It is critical that the person acknowledges and validates his or her suffering, resists the societal dominant narratives about post-loss (e.g. being a victim, having PTSD) and learns to rebuild the life story, the narrative.

Clinical methods – examples to try

There are many different ways of achieving an effective narrative that incorporates post-traumatic growth. The methods we have discussed previously are all helpful, but here we provide examples – related examples – of how you might be able to begin to develop growth.

A therapeutic journal

In its simplest terms, this is a journal in which you write about your traumatic experiences, your reactions and your thoughts. It is an ongoing process, where you record your everyday dealings with people, your current thoughts about events, your work or social life, where you think these have been affected by your traumatic experiences. You do need somewhere quiet to write, somewhere you can reflect. The content of the journal is yours to do with as you wish. No one has to read it. At first, it is probably better that no one does read it; it is your interpretation of thoughts, feelings and behaviour. Begin with an account of the traumatic experience and your reactions to it (in a similar way to that discussed in Chapter 6). This may take you several days or even weeks, but it will enable you to create a detailed account. Once this is completed, move on to the next stage, that of writing about your everyday life and how it is affected by your traumatic experiences. Be as honest and detailed as possible. It may be that you feel your relationship with your husband or wife is affected by something you said or did; put it in and try to explain it. Perhaps it is your reaction to something a work colleague did; put it in and try to explain it. Over time, you can look back at your account and hopefully start to see patterns in the behaviour and the reactions. This may help you to start thinking about how you behave, or how you think, or why you react emotionally the way you do. Is there something about certain people who seem to react badly to you? Can you explain to them what you are feeling? Again, there are no hard-and-fast rules, and this is not meant to be an easy process. And it will only work if you can sit and write for longish periods on a regular basis. It is not for everyone.

The Pennebaker process

James Pennebaker has developed a simpler approach to writing about traumatic experiences. He argues (and there is some evidence for his claim) that writing deeply and consistently about traumatic experiences has clear mental and possibly physical health benefits. Pennebaker argues that writing about the worst aspects of the trauma for a period of 20–30 minutes a day for three days will lead to positive change. Write in a similar way to the above, but focus on the worst aspects of the traumatic event and your responses.

Oral narrative approaches

Many people do not enjoy writing but would prefer to present their thoughts by speaking. The oral tradition is as old as humanity. In pre-literate societies it was (and is) very common for people to learn tales by heart and repeat them to suitable audiences. Oral approaches take many forms, but if you do not want other people to listen to what you have to say at this point then it is valuable to record your thoughts continually over a period of days or weeks. These can then be played back, and you can develop and add to these thoughts in the same way as with writing. Having the record, whether it is oral or written, is very helpful, as you can see what you were thinking in the past, and you can spend time developing these thoughts rather than try to solve all your major problems in one session.

These narrative approaches really do help in the development of meaning after a traumatic event; they do help you to develop in a positive manner, to come to terms with the traumatic experience and to learn from it – in other words, to experience growth.

Summary

Post-traumatic growth is more than engaging in non-negative thinking. It is not just about trying to deal with your traumatic memories. It is about positive change as a result of dealing with your experiences. It is related to psychological well-being, to physical and mental health; it is related to developing the meaning of life, having good relationships with others, and being satisfied with your life.

Having said that, a word of caution. Throughout this book we have stressed how complicated the reactions to traumatic events are. Experiencing post-traumatic growth does not mean that you are not still traumatized. There is a sense in which growth and trauma are different aspects of experience rather than different ends of a spectrum; it is perfectly possible, and indeed common, for people to experience both PTSD and growth at the same time.

10

What professional help is available?

This has been discussed to some extent in the treatment chapters. Here, we discuss the range of help that is available, along with specific addresses of where to obtain such help. The help ranges from information sources, such as this book, to obtaining a referral from your GP to specialist help from clinical psychologists, psychiatrists and other mental health workers, through to the help provided by charities such as – for armed forces veterans – the Royal British Legion and Combat Stress. Other charities such as the Samaritans may also be helpful. A guide such as this can never be comprehensive, and books and websites do go out of date. There are also issues about the availability of particular sources in different countries. This is why we have listed some of the general sources of help that are available.

The chapter is split into several sections: professional therapists, charities and websites. There are many books available about trauma and PTSD, and a selection of these is listed in Further reading, along with a number of films that have portrayed trauma.

Professional therapists

As we have discussed to some extent in earlier chapters, there is a range of professional help available in the UK; some of these are paralleled in other countries, or there may be similar kinds of help available. The process of seeking help will differ according to country. Here we discuss the UK.

It is normal practice in the UK for someone seeking help with a mental health issue such as trauma to visit the GP first of all and be referred to an appropriate mental health specialist. There are a number of these available. Though practice and availability does vary to some extent around the country, there are the following key groups:

Clinical psychologists

These are, for many people, the best option, as they are fully trained to use a range of therapies (although they cannot prescribe drugs), and you can be referred to one by your GP. Their background is in psychology, with a psychology first degree and then a clinical doctorate, making six years of psychology training. They usually have a broad range of experience treating the full range of mental health disorders in different groups, though they may, after training, specialize in specific areas. While many clinical psychologists are employed by the NHS, many also practise privately. For trauma patients, the problem can be the waiting list, which is often months (sometimes years) long for treatment on the NHS, and trauma can often get worse if left untreated. As with so many things, if you can afford it you can be treated privately much more quickly. Clinical psychologists are chartered by the British Psychological Society (BPS) – though this may change in the next few years – and the BPS website provides details of practitioners in your area.

Psychiatrists

Psychiatrists are fully trained medical practitioners who, after qualifying as medical doctors, have specialized in mental health. They are usually trained to use a range of psychological therapies, and they can also prescribe drugs. You can be referred to a psychiatrist by your GP. Sometimes, clinical psychologists and psychiatrists will work together on a case, with the psychiatrist taking responsibility for any drug treatment and the clinical psychologist undertaking the psychotherapy. Psychiatrists are members of the British Medical Association, which can provide details of local psychiatrists.

Cognitive behavioural therapists

There are many kinds of CBT practitioners available around the country; some work within the NHS, some work privately and others work for specific charities. For a list of qualified CBT practitioners in your area, you should go to the BABCP website, which provides full details.

Counsellors

Counsellors are increasingly used within the NHS to provide support for mental health disorders. Many GP surgeries now make use of a counsellor for one or more sessions a week. Normally, a counsellor is less well trained in psychological therapy and may be less suitable for dealing with trauma cases, but counsellors do come from a variety of backgrounds with a wide range of training, so it is worth finding out about any that are available near you. Counsellors can also be found in private practice and work in the charity sector. If your case relates to a specific area, for example breast cancer, then you may find a breast cancer charity that provides helpful counselling. The British Association of Counselling and Psychotherapy can provide details of counsellors in your area.

Psychoanalysts

For those who prefer to be treated psychoanalytically, there are psychoanalysts available around the country. These are less likely to be available on the NHS, though you should ask your GP. Psychoanalysts receive a number of years' training in psychoanalysis, which usually involves them undergoing psychoanalysis as part of their treatment. The Institute of Psychoanalysis can provide details of practitioners in your area.

Other available therapies

Recently, the NHS has started providing more therapists who specialize in basic CBT and a number of other therapies, including the provision of self-help books and other guidance (part of the Improving Access to Psychotherapy programme). These are unlikely to be suitable in serious cases, though they may be of some help. Again, you can be referred by your GP.

Charities

There are many charities that work in areas relating to PTSD and trauma. Most are specific to a particular kind of traumatic event, such as rape or war.

Combat Stress

Combat Stress was set up after the First World War in order to help veterans who experience mental health disorders as a result of their experiences of war. It has a network of welfare officers around the country (who are themselves ex-forces) and residential accommodation for people who need it. It provides a lot of the expert treatment that is necessary for war veterans. It is funded partly by the MoD, partly by the NHS (who refer people to the charity) and partly by donations.

Royal British Legion

Again, this was set up after the First World War to look after ex-services personnel, not just regarding mental health issues but providing more general support. The Royal British Legion does provide some help for veterans experiencing mental health issues, particularly for families in need.

For details of these and other helpful charities, see Useful addresses.

Websites

If you want to find out information about a particular kind of traumatic event, or get involved with online discussions, there are numerous websites available. Some people appear to benefit from the ability to discuss their situation anonymously at an online forum, though you do need to be careful, as the identity of people is rarely verified. You may not be communicating with the person you think you are communicating with.

Websites vary in their usefulness and accuracy. Again without being comprehensive, in Useful addresses we list a few that are very helpful and which themselves can lead you to further information sources.

11

Conclusions

This final brief chapter draws together the key points made throughout the book, showing that we have a good – if still imperfect – understanding of traumatic stress. We know something about its causes and effects, and the range of symptoms people experience, and we have some therapies that work very well for some people – but unfortunately not for everyone. This chapter also provides some advice on what you can do to help yourself, now that you know something more about the issues.

Traumatic events

Traumatic events take many forms, and something that is traumatic for one person is not for another; this is why both the event itself and the symptoms afterwards are required before one can get a diagnosis of PTSD. Traumatic events include the experience of war (either as a soldier or as a civilian), becoming a refugee, rape or sexual abuse, natural or manmade disasters, car accidents or the unexpected death of a loved one; but there are many other events that may also be classified as traumatic. They can also be either single incidents, such as a case of rape or a disaster, or they can be complex events such as war or prolonged sexual abuse. People do respond differently to these cases. Complex PTSD, which may arise from prolonged exposure to traumatic events, can be more difficult to deal with and treat than simple PTSD resulting from a single event.

We must also think about the limitations of traumatic events. While the event was initially described as something 'outside the range of normal human experience', it was quickly realized that most people experience traumatic events at some point in their lives, but they do not necessarily – or even usually – have serious psychological consequences. It is debatable whether the death of a loved one is traumatic. It may well be if the person is unexpectedly killed next to you, but it is not traumatic when, for example, a grandparent dies at a very old age. We should not confuse trauma and grief, though some of the symptoms may be similar. Also, you are not traumatized by the sight of a terrible event on television, though it may be extremely upsetting. The term 'trauma' has become used too widely, and in so doing it loses some of its meaning. Here we are interested in genuinely traumatic events, where a person's life, or that of a loved one, is seriously threatened. There are several dangers in overusing the term 'trauma'. Genuinely traumatized people may not be easily identified; saying, for example, that the death of a pet is traumatic is unhelpful when considering the impact of a genuine traumatic experience. The death of a pet can be very upsetting, but it is not traumatic.

There is a further complication with pathologizing the idea of trauma. We know from evidence during the World Wars that someone with a mental disturbance who thinks he or she is genuinely ill may well become a casualty, and it is very difficult to get better again. Instead, it is often more appropriate to think of the response to trauma as being a normal response to an extraordinary situation, with the view that one will begin to forget and will get better over time. Of course, in order to receive treatment a person must have a diagnosable disorder, which brings us back to whether or not mental disorders should be classified in the same way as physical disorders, particularly when, as in the case of trauma, the response is not unexpected given the extremely stressful situation the person has been through. This debate rages in academia and across therapeutic networks, and is unlikely to be resolved in the near future. For now, we can say that, where possible, it is better not to be labelled with a disorder. The experience of traumatic symptoms is a normal reaction to an abnormal life-threatening event, and not necessarily pathological. It becomes pathological when it goes on for a substantial period of time, and significantly affects your family, social or occupational life.

When people go through traumatic events and are not traumatized, it does not mean they do not experience the same symptoms as PTSD, but that the symptoms are temporary, and perhaps last for days or weeks. It is normal to be very upset after a traumatic incident which is, by definition, life-threatening. It is normal to experience some symptoms, just as it is normal to experience no symptoms at all.

Shared suffering

If you are traumatized it is important to remember, even if you do not feel it is doing you any good, that you are not alone. There are many people who have very severe reactions relating to trauma, and even though it can feel at times that you are suffering more than anyone, there are others who are sharing a similar response. Having said that, we do know that most people do recover, one way or another.

Common symptoms

As we have said repeatedly, traumatic stress is a complex disorder and people respond in very different ways, but there are a number of things that seem to happen to most people who are traumatized. The key symptoms that most people experience are:

- traumatic memories, which may take the form of nightmares, flashbacks, or the inability to get things out of your head;
- avoidance of things that remind you of the traumatic event, usually to avoid the emotions and memories associated with reminders;

- emotional numbing, the inability to experience normal emotions;
- physiological hyperarousal (the inability to concentrate or attend to tasks normally) or an exaggerated startle response.

It is also common for people to experience other symptoms, such as:

- depression
- generalized anxiety
- substance abuse, such as drinking too much or taking illegal drugs
- unmanageable anger, often against the self or family members.

Traumatized people often have what we call dissociation: that is, parts of their memories are separated from other parts, and they find it difficult to put these pieces back together in a way that makes sense. This is related to a problem with putting memories where they belong – in the past, rather than constantly being in consciousness – or there may be either a deliberate or an unconscious lack of remembering key elements of the traumatic incident.

Treatment

As we have discussed, there are a number of ways in which the symptoms of trauma can be treated. The evidence points to CBT and EMDR as being particularly effective treatments, though the use of drugs is sometimes necessary and helpful in reducing symptoms. Nevertheless, no single treatment is ideal for everyone. Most of the talking therapies require you to be willing, able and motivated to talk deeply about what happened to you and what effects it has had on your life. For that reason alone, they are not suited to everyone. Many people are unwilling or unable to talk about their experiences and memories. Furthermore, just because the evidence for CBT and EMDR is better than for other talking therapies, that does not mean that a different approach would not be more suitable and more effective for you. It is a matter of finding the right approach for each individual, and we hope that this book has gone some way to helping you with those choices. The Further reading section at the end of the book will help you find more information about the therapies.

Narrative development

Throughout the book we have argued that the key element in learning to deal with traumatic events is the development of a narrative, the ability to integrate the event and its consequences into your own life story or autobiography. Most trauma researchers and therapists would agree that traumatic events lead to a breakdown of the self, of the life story, of the way we think about ourselves. Most therapy is about rebuilding that story, sometimes explicitly so, as in the case of narrative therapy, sometimes more implicitly, as with CBT, which focuses on key elements, such as learning to relax or helping to change erroneous beliefs, and coming to accept the person you are (or have become).

In this way, therapy is more than just building a narrative. Where people are anxious or frightened, it is important to help them learn skills to deal with their anxiety. This is where CBT has an advantage over other forms of therapy, in that it explicitly teaches skills such as relaxation relating specifically to the anxiety-inducing stimulus. The cognitive component of CBT is designed to help people make sense of their narrative, their life story. By helping people to realize that their belief systems are not working properly, and helping them to examine the way they think about other people and the world, the therapist is taking the first stages along the development of the narrative, explicitly helping individuals to make sense of their experiences.

We discussed how methods of storytelling, of repeating the

traumatic memory several – sometimes many – times, complete with details of associated emotions and behaviours, are likely, over time, to lead to a reduction in the anxiety that is felt when recalling the traumatic memory, so having genuine benefits. Many narratives are produced after a war; whether these are as films, books, plays or poems, or whether they are unpublished journals or stories, there seems to be a need among many people to tell their story of the traumatic experience that is war.

Legal implications of traumatic stress

As it is an accepted diagnostic category, the construct of PTSD is used widely in law. There are increasing numbers of legal cases relating to traumatic stress. This area is controversial, partly because of the difficulties of finding the appropriate cut-off points where one person is classified as traumatized and another is not. Expert opinion (that of clinical psychologists and psychiatrists) regarding particular cases can differ markedly. One expert may argue in court that a person is unable to work because of his or her traumatic experiences, and another may argue that the same person's ability to work is unaffected. Under British law, it can be difficult for traumatized people to deal with the arguments that can ensue in the court situation, possibly making things worse. There are arguments about whether someone should receive compensation for traumatic stress, and if so, how much. Veterans of the Second World War may become upset when they see recent cases of trauma receiving hundreds of thousands of pounds for a single experience, while they have been having similar experiences for years. It is very difficult to be fair.

Another serious legal issue for trauma cases is coming before the court as a witness. Someone who has been raped may not wish to undergo what can be a very difficult cross-examination in court, involving presenting all the details of the rape to an open court. Even if a dispensation is allowed so that evidence can be presented in camera, this is still difficult – and then of course this may be jeopardizing the defendant's position, as the defendant's barrister may not be able to carry out a full cross-examination.

It is possible for a diagnosis of PTSD to help people who are imprisoned. In the case of 12 people locked up without charge or trial in Belmarsh Prison in London because it was thought they were potential terrorists, a diagnosis of PTSD was made on the basis that the PTSD was caused by the imprisonment itself. It was successfully argued by a team of clinical psychologists and psychiatrists that locking people up without any indication of whether they would be released, and with no opportunity to defend themselves in a trial, was a traumatic stressor which led directly to PTSD. In this case, the construct of PTSD was being used politically, in order to obtain justice.

Traumatic experiences as permanent change

The aim of therapy is not to help people become as they were before their traumatic experience, but to help them learn to deal with their memories and emotions in ways that are effective and to make sense of the post-trauma world. That may be as simple as providing skills to deal with anxiety, or it may relate to more complex meaning-making or life story development. It is sometimes easier to think of trauma not as an illness but as part of life's course (most of us experience traumatic events at some point in our lives, though for some it is much worse than others), and as part of our development as human beings. Such experiences help us to know ourselves better, and to emerge stronger from such experiences.

The more you know about the symptoms of trauma, the better. As you start on the road to recovery, the more you understand, the more you are able to deal with the memories, and the greater the possibility of emerging from the experience stronger, with a better understanding of your life. The key existential question asks what is the meaning of life. If traumatic experiences have any benefits – and that is certainly arguable – then it may be that they can help us think about what life means to us, and to develop a greater understanding of life and death.

Appendix: Self-report measures

The following measures are designed to give you some idea of the extent of your symptoms and how they change over time. These measures are not intended to be a substitute for a full assessment for any of the disorders, but simply provide an indication of whether you may have a disorder. Only a fully qualified practitioner (e.g. a clinical psychologist or psychiatrist) can determine whether there is a diagnosis of the disorder. The measures for PTSD, depression, generalized anxiety and substance abuse relate to the diagnostic criteria for those disorders. They are not reliable and valid standardized scales. If you need further information about whether or not you may have these disorders, please see your medical practitioner.

The measures for PTSD, depression, anxiety and substance abuse are based on *DSM* criteria, and provide a general indication of whether or not you have a particular disorder. The measure for coping is to help you see which kinds of coping strategies you normally use.

Please answer the measures honestly.

Measure 1: Post-traumatic stress disorder

Criterion A: The stressor

1	Have you experienced, witnessed, or been confronted with an event or events that involve actual or threatened death or serious injury, or a threat to the physical integrity of yourself or others?	YES	NO
2	Did your response involve intense fear, helplessness or horror? Note: in children, this may be expressed instead by disorganized or agitated behaviour	YES	NO

Criterion B: Intrusive recollection
Do you experience any of the following?

3 Recurrent and intrusive distressing recollections   YES   NO
of the event, including images, thoughts or
perceptions (note: in young children, repetitive
play may occur in which themes or aspects of the
trauma are expressed)

4 Recurrent distressing dreams of the event (note: in   YES   NO
children, there may be frightening dreams without
recognizable content)

5 Acting or feeling as if the traumatic event   YES   NO
were recurring, such as a sense of reliving the
experience, illusions, hallucinations and dissociative
flashback episodes, including any that occur upon
awakening or when intoxicated (note: in children,
trauma-specific re-enactment may occur)

6 Intense psychological distress at exposure to   YES   NO
internal or external cues that symbolize or
resemble an aspect of the traumatic event

7 Physiological reactions when exposed to internal or   YES   NO
external cues that remind you of an aspect of the
traumatic event

Criterion C: Avoidance or numbing
Do you experience any of the following?

8 Efforts to avoid thoughts, feelings or conversations   YES   NO
associated with the trauma

9 Efforts to avoid activities, places or people that   YES   NO
arouse recollections of the trauma

10 Inability to recall an important aspect of the   YES   NO
trauma

11 Markedly diminished interest or participation in   YES   NO
significant activities

12 Feeling of detachment or estrangement from others   YES   NO

13	Restricted range of emotions (e.g. unable to have loving feelings)	YES	NO
14	Sense of foreshortened future (e.g. 'I do not expect to have a career, marriage, children, a normal life span . . .')	YES	NO

Criterion D: Hyperarousal
Do you experience any of the following?

15	Difficulty falling or staying asleep	YES	NO
16	Irritability or outbursts of anger	YES	NO
17	Difficulty concentrating	YES	NO
18	Hyper-vigilance	YES	NO
19	Exaggerated startle response	YES	NO

Criterion E: Duration

20	Have you experienced the symptoms described in Criteria B, C and D for more than one month?	YES	NO

Criterion F: Functional significance

21	Have your symptoms caused significant distress or impairment to your social, occupational or other important areas of functioning?	YES	NO

Specify whether
Acute: if duration of symptoms is less than three months
Chronic: if duration of symptoms is three months or more
With or without delayed onset: onset of symptoms at least six months after the stressor

Scoring

Criterion A: You must have answered YES to both question 1 and question 2.

Criterion B: You must have answered YES to at least one of questions 3–7.

Criterion C: You must have answered YES to at least three of questions 8–14.

Criterion D: You must have answered YES to at least two of questions 15–19.

Criterion E: You must have answered YES to question 20.

Criterion F: You must have answered YES to question 21.

If you have answered YES as indicated above for Criteria A–F then you may have PTSD. You can also see whether it is acute, chronic or delayed onset.

As already indicated, self-report is unreliable and you will need to obtain an accurate diagnosis from a medical practitioner.

Measure 2: Depression

There are many types of depression, and varying degrees of severity. The diagnostic indicator provided below is only for your information, and does not indicate with certainty whether you have clinical depression, nor does it cover the range of different types of depression.

Please indicate which of the following you have experienced during the same two-week period, and which represent a change from previous functioning (do not count those relating to another physical health disorder). This can be scored either by the person or by someone who observed the person regularly

Criterion A

1	Depressed mood most of the day, nearly every day, e.g. feeling sad or tearful (note: in children and adolescents, can be irritable mood)	YES	NO
2	Markedly diminished interest or pleasure in all, or almost all, activities most of the day, nearly every day	YES	NO
3	Significant weight loss when not dieting or weight gain (e.g. a change of more than 5 per cent of body weight in a month), or decrease or increase in appetite nearly every day (note: in children, consider failure to make expected weight gains)	YES	NO

4	Sleeping too little or too much nearly every day	YES	NO
5	Physical agitation or unusual physical movements nearly every day	YES	NO
6	Fatigue or loss of energy nearly every day	YES	NO
7	Feelings of worthlessness or excessive or inappropriate guilt (which may be delusional) nearly every day (not merely self-reproach or guilt about being ill)	YES	NO
8	Diminished ability to think or concentrate, or indecisiveness, nearly every day	YES	NO
9	Recurrent thoughts of death (not just fear of dying), recurrent thoughts of suicide without a specific plan, or a suicide attempt or a specific plan for committing suicide	YES	NO

Criterion B

Do the symptoms cause clinically significant distress or impairment in social, occupational, or other important areas of functioning?   YES   NO

Criterion C

Are the symptoms due to the direct physiological effects of a substance (e.g. a drug of abuse, a medication) or a general medical condition (e.g. hypothyroidism)?   YES   NO

Interpretation

In order to be classified as having depression, you should have answered YES to five or more questions in Criterion A, including either (1) depressed mood or (2) loss of interest or pleasure, YES to Criterion B and NO to Criterion C.

Measure 3: Anxiety

1 Do you have excessive anxiety about a number of events or activities, occurring more days than not, for at least six months?   YES   NO

2 Do you find it difficult to control that worry?   YES   NO

3 Is the anxiety and worry associated with the following:

   (a) restlessness or feeling keyed up or on edge?   YES   NO

   (b) being easily fatigued?   YES   NO

   (c) difficulty concentrating or mind going blank?   YES   NO

   (d) irritability?   YES   NO

   (e) muscle tension?   YES   NO

   (f) sleep disturbance?   YES   NO

4 Is the anxiety about a specific problem, for instance, social phobia, gaining weight or a serious illness?   YES   NO

5 Does the anxiety cause significant distress or impairment in your social or work life?   YES   NO

6   Does the anxiety occur specifically during events such as alcohol use or as part of a medical condition?   YES   NO

Interpretation
In order to be classified as having generalized anxiety disorder, you should have answered YES to questions 1 and 2, YES to at least three of the question 3 answers, NO to question 4, YES to question 5, and NO to question 6.

Measure 4: Substance abuse (e.g. alcohol, illegal drugs)

Have the following occurred over the last 12 months?

1   Recurrent substance use resulting in a failure to fulfil your major work or social obligations (e.g. absence from work or school)   YES   NO

2   Recurrent substance use in situations that are dangerous (e.g. driving a car)   YES   NO

3   Recurrent substance use resulting in legal problems (e.g. being arrested or charged with offences)   YES   NO

4   Continued substance use despite having social or personal problems relating to the substance use   YES   NO

Interpretation
In order to be classified as having substance abuse you need to answer YES to all four questions.

Useful addresses

Therapy information

Your first port of call for therapy is usually your GP. But it can help to learn something about the different therapies that are available.

The Association for Counselling and Psychotherapy Online
Website: www.acto-uk.org
This provides details of practitioners who provide online therapy.

The British Association for Behavioural and Cognitive Psychotherapies
Tel.: 0161 797 4484
Website: www.babcp.com
The main organization dealing with practitioners of cognitive behaviour therapy, and providing accreditation.

The British Association of Counselling and Psychotherapy
Tel.: 01455 883316 (help and information for choosing a counsellor)
Website: www.bacp.co.uk
This association represents many counsellors and psychotherapists across the UK; phone for help and information in choosing one in a convenient locality.

The British Medical Association
Tel.: 020 7387 4499
Website: www.bma.org.uk
The doctors' professional organization.

The British Psychological Society
Tel.: 0116 254 9568
Website: www.bps.org.uk
The key organization for psychologists in the UK. Here you will find details of clinical psychologists and others interested in traumatic stress.

Combat Stress
Tel.: 01372 841600
Website: ww.combatstress.org.uk
A charity delivering specialist, trauma-focused treatment to ex-service men and women and to their families.

Eye Movement Desensitization and Reprocessing (EMDR) Association
Website: www.emdrassociation.org.uk
EMDR is a form of psychotherapy developed in the 1980s to help resolve symptoms arising from disturbing life experiences. The website provides details about EMDR and practitioners of this specific discipline.

The Institute of Psychoanalysis
Tel.: 020 7563 5002 (London Clinic)
Website: www.psychoanalysis.org.uk
For those who are interested in psychoanalytic treatment.

General information

David Baldwin's Trauma Pages
Website: www.trauma-pages.com
David Baldwin, a licensed psychologist practising in Oregon, specializes in treating PTSD. His site contains details of articles, resources, general information and links to help with and support those who have experienced a variety of situations that have led to traumatic stress.

European Society for Traumatic Stress Studies
Website: www.estss.org
Based in the Netherlands, the society brings together practitioners and researchers in the area of traumatic stress.

International Society for Traumatic Stress Studies
Website: www.istss.org
This international professional membership organization promotes the advancement and exchange of knowledge about severe stress and trauma. Its headquarters are in Deerfield, Illinois.

National Center for Post-Traumatic Stress Disorder
Website: www.ptsd.va.gov
This centre is run by the US Department of Veterans' Affairs and they publish the PILOTS database, which lists the scientific publications relating to PTSD. The website gives advice about PTSD and links to other organizations that will help.

Royal British Legion
Tel.: 020 3207 2100
Website: www.britishlegion.org.uk

World Health Organization
Website: www.who.int/en
Provides useful information about general health, including PTSD.

Other organizations

Addaction
Website: www.addaction.org.uk
Provides help for people with drug problems.

Alcohol Issues
Website: www.alcoholissues.co.uk
An organization that will help with problems relating to alcohol.

Relate
Tel.: 0300 100 1234
Website: www.relate.org,.uk
This charity deals with issues concerning relationships.

Samaritans
Tel.: 08457 909090
Website: www.samaritans.org
Provides confidential, non-judgemental emotional support for people who are experiencing feelings of distress.

Victim Support
Tel. (Supportline): 0845 30 30 900
Website: www.victimsupport.org.uk
A charity which provides assistance to people who are the victims of crime.

Further reading, films and plays

Books about PTSD and trauma

There are many books published about traumatic stress, some for academics, some for clinicians, and others for members of the general public. Here are just a few to get you started.

Bartlett, F., *Remembering: A study in experimental and social psychology.* Cambridge University Press, Cambridge, 1932.

Bremner, J. D., *Does Stress Damage the Brain?* W.W. Norton, New York, 2005.

Calhoun, L. and Tedeschi, R. (eds), *Handbook of Posttraumatic Growth.* Lawrence Erlbaum, New York, 2006.

Creamer, M., 'A cognitive processing formulation of posttrauma reactions'. In Kleber, R., Figley, C., and Gersons, B., (eds), *Beyond Trauma: Cultural and societal dynamics.* Plenum, New York, 1995.

Foa, E., Keane, T. and Friedman, M. (eds), *Effective Treatments for PTSD.* Guilford Press, New York, 2000.

Harvey, J. and Pauwels, B. (eds), *Post-Traumatic Stress Theory.* Brunner/Mazel, New York, 2000.

Herman, J., *Trauma and Recovery.* Basic Books, New York, 1992.

Janet, P., *Psychological Healing.* Allen & Unwin, Oxford, 1926.

Joseph, S. and Linley, A., *Trauma, Recovery and Growth: Positive psychological perspectives on post-traumatic stress.* Wiley, London, 2008.

Joseph, S., Williams, R. and Yule, W., *Understanding Post Traumatic Stress: A psychosocial perspective on PTSD and treatment.* John Wiley & Sons, Chichester, 1997.

Neimeyer, R., 'Restorying loss: fostering growth in the posttraumatic narrative'. In Calhoun, L. and Tedeschi, R. (eds), *Handbook of Posttraumatic Growth: Research and practice.* Lawrence Erlbaum, London, 2006.

Pennebaker, J. (2004), *Writing to Heal: A guided journal for recovering from trauma and emotional upheaval.* New Harbinger Publications, Oakland, 2004.

Resick, P., *Stress and Trauma.* Psychology Press, London, 2001.

Schauer, M., Neuner, F. and Elbert, T., *Narrative Exposure Therapy: A short term intervention for traumatic stress disorders after war, terror or torture.* Hogrefe & Huber, Göttingen, 2004.

Scott, M., *Moving On After Trauma.* Routledge, London, 2007.

Shapiro, F., *Eye Movement Desensitisation and Reprocessing: Basic principles, protocols and procedures.* Guilford Press, London, 2001.

Yule, W. (ed.), *Post-Traumatic Stress Disorders.* John Wiley & Sons, Chichester, 1999.

Other books and poetry

The list that follows includes books and poetry written by people who have survived traumatic experiences, and also books by people who have not experienced trauma but have tried to represent trauma through fiction. The amount of literature generated shows the importance of people wanting to present their narratives of trauma – not just their own individual experiences but the social and cultural experiences of the many millions of people who have lived through the traumatic twentieth century and beyond. Every war seems to generate its own literature, both autobiographical and fictional.

As discussed in Chapter 1, we can go right back to Ancient Greece to find examples of traumatic stress. Homer's *Iliad* is a good example of war trauma. Some of the great novelists of the nineteenth century wrote about wartime experiences: Tolstoy's account of fighting in the Crimean War, for instance, or his *War and Peace*, an account of the Napoleonic Wars; and Zola's account of the Franco-Prussian War.

The First World War generated a lot of literature, including Erich Maria Remarque's *All Quiet on the Western Front*, Ernst Jünger's *Storm of Steel*, Ernest Hemingway's *A Farewell to Arms*, Siegfried Sassoon's *Memoirs of an Infantry Officer* and Vera Brittain's *Testament of Youth*. The writing of the war poets, Wilfred Owen, Siegfried Sassoon and others, represents the nature of war as experienced in the trenches of the First World War. Later fiction about that war includes the *Regeneration* trilogy by Pat Barker and Sebastian Faulks' *Birdsong*.

The Second World War generated even more literature, including a great deal of writing about the Holocaust, for example the work of Primo Levi and Anne Frank. Guy Sajer wrote *The Forgotten Soldier* about the Russian Front. The suffering of Berliners, particularly at the end of the war, has been described by Cornelius Ryan (*The Last Battle*), Antony Beevor (*Berlin: The downfall, 1945*) and, from the personal perspective, by the anonymous author of *A Woman in Berlin*.

Solzhenitsyn wrote about the trauma in Russia during much of the twentieth century, particularly the Soviet years, including his account of the Gulags, *The Gulag Archipelago*.

In more recent times, there have been accounts from wars such as Vietnam (Bao Ninh's *The Sorrow of War*) and Bosnia (e.g. *Zlata's Diary: A child's life in Sarajevo* by Zlata Filipović and *Not My Turn to Die: Memoirs of a broken childhood in Bosnia* by Savo Heleta).

There are also many narrative accounts of other traumatic experiences such as child abuse and rape (such as *I Never Told Anyone: Writings by women survivors of child abuse* edited by Ellen Bass and Louise Thornton, *Don't Tell Mummy: A true story of the ultimate betrayal* by Toni Maguire, and *After Silence: Rape and my journey back* by Nancy Venable Raine).

Films, plays and TV

There are very many films and plays about traumatic experiences, the earliest film probably being *All Quiet on the Western Front* (1934). The Second World War led to many films and a good number of these describe trauma, particularly when representing the Holocaust, e.g. *Shoah*. Then there is *M*A*S*H**, which satirically examines trauma in the Korean War, through the Oliver Stone films about the Vietnam War (*Platoon, Born on the Fourth of July, Heaven and Earth*) to films about Bosnia (such as *No Man's Land, Welcome to Sarajevo*, Peter Kosminsky's *Warriors* and *Pretty Village, Pretty Flame*), all of which display the brutalizing effect of war. There are also many films and TV documentaries about the trauma associated with the Iraq and Afghanistan Wars.

Finally, as always, Shakespeare has described personal experience in great detail. In *Henry IV Part I*, Lady Percy worries about her husband, who clearly has symptoms of traumatic stress:

Lady Percy	Trauma symptom
O, my good lord, why are you thus alone?	Social withdrawal
For what offence have I this fortnight been	
A banish'd woman from my Harry's bed?	Sexual dysfunction
Tell me, sweet lord, what is't that takes from thee	Lack of interest in ordinary
Thy stomach, pleasure and thy golden sleep?	things such as food
Why dost thou bend thine eyes upon the earth	Depressed, startle
And start so often when thou sit'st alone?	response
Why hast thou lost the fresh blood in thy cheeks,	
And given my treasures and my rights of thee	Somatic symptoms,
To thick-ey'd musing, and curs'd melancholy?	depression
In thy faint slumbers I by thee have watch'd,	
And heard thee murmur tales of iron wars,	Nightmares, bad dreams
Speak terms of manage to thy bounding steed;	
Cry 'Courage! To the field!' And thou hast talked	
Of sallies and retires, of trenches, tents,	
Of palisadoes, frontiers, parapets,	
Of basilisks, of cannon, culverin,	
Of prisoners' ransom, and of soldiers slain	
And all the currents of a heady fight.	
Thy spirit within thee hast been so at war	Upset, anxious, sleep
And thus hath so bestirr'd thee in thy sleep,	problems
That beads of sweat have stood upon thy brow	
Like bubbles in a late-disturbed stream;	Physiological reactions
And in thy face strange motions have appeared,	
Such as we see when men restrain their breath	
On some great sudden hest. O, what portents	Worry for the future
are these?	
Some heavy business hath my lord in hand,	Loved ones worried
And I must know it, else he loves me not.	about relationship

Index